Growing Up With Epilepsy

GROWING UP
WITH EPILEPSY

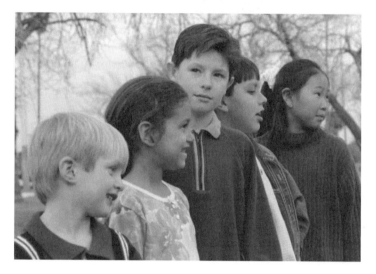

A PRACTICAL GUIDE FOR PARENTS

Lynn Bennett Blackburn, Ph.D.

Demos

DEMOS MEDICAL PUBLISHING, 386 PARK AVENUE SOUTH, NEW YORK, NEW YORK 10016

Library of Congress Cataloging-in-Publication Data

Blackburn, Lynn Bennett.
   Growing up with epilepsy : a practical guide for parents / Lynn Bennett Blackburn.
   p. cm.
Includes bibliographical references.
   ISBN 1-888799-74-9 (pbk.)
   1. Epilepsy in children—Popular works. I. Title.
   RJ496.E6 B534 2002
   618.92'853—dc21
                              2002015587

Printed in Canada

Dedication

To every child who,
as Bethany said,
has "too much 'lectricity"
in his or her head.

Acknowledgment

THIS BOOK IS THE RESULT of four key elements: inspiration, time, support, and good editing. Inspiration for this book came from the many families with whom I have had the privilege of working. Over the years, I have rejoiced with them in the joy of a successful medical intervention, marveled at their creativity in managing the complications that epilepsy created in their lives, and been impressed by their perseverance in dealing with schools to make sure that their child's needs are met. I thank each of these families for allowing me to be a small part of their lives. Inspiration for the book also came from the dedicated epilepsy treatment teams with whom I have had the pleasure to work. I thank each of these physicians, nurses, and EEG techs for the contributions they have made to my understanding of the management of epilepsy.

To have the time necessary to complete this project, the administration at St. Louis Children's Hospital and the Psychology Department allowed me to reduce my hours at the hospital. I thank Dr. Russell Hoffmann, who worked with administration to make this happen. I thank my wonderful colleagues, Dr. Tara Spevack and Dr. Steve Kanne, for their support. I always knew the services I cover were in their good hands on my day away from the hospital.

The third key in creating a book is emotional support. I am deeply indebted to my husband, Richard. Over the past 28 years, his belief in me has provided me with the basis for attempting new things. You can take risks in life when you know that you can always find unconditional love waiting for you at home.

The final element in creating a book is a good editor. I am grateful to Tammy Chajon for taking the time to read each chapter. Having no background in epilepsy, she made sure that I hadn't slipped into neuropsychological jargon, medical jargon, or assumed information that a parent may not have. I thank the staff at Demos Medical Publishing for their great suggestions, helpful editing, and finishing touches.

Contents

Preface

WHEN YOU BUY A NEW CAR, it comes with an owner's manual. At least once in their child's life, every parent has wished that their child came with a similar manual. In place of an owner's manual, parents talk to friends or seek guidance from their own parents. When your child has epilepsy, this informal network fails. Friends and family members often lack the experience necessary to be helpful. The goal of *Growing Up with Epilepsy* is to provide you with an owner's manual to negotiate the unique challenges of childhood epilepsy.

The unpredictability of seizures and the potential side effects of medication often result in confusion about what is fair to expect for the child with epilepsy. Confronting misunderstanding from others leaves you in the role of epilepsy educator, a role that you may feel ill-prepared to undertake. Each stage in your child's life provides unique issues to address, issues ranging from finding day care to school programming to driving. Children with epilepsy can grow into independent, effective adults. To do this, they need discipline to build appropriate behavior, social skills so that they will be accepted, and the educational background that provides the basis for eventual employment. This book provides you with the tools to discipline your child, to support social development, and to negotiate the educational system, making you an effective advocate for your child.

In my 20 years of working with children with epilepsy, I am continually impressed by the fact that no two children with epilepsy are the same. Each child and each family presents unique needs. Because of this, I work with a team. The unique talents of each team member let us, as a group, meet the unique needs of each patient. In addition to providing you with basic tools, *Growing Up with Epilepsy* identifies resources, places you can contact, additional materials you can read, and the kinds of professionals in your community who may help you and your child. The goal of *Growing Up with Epilepsy* is to help you build the resource team for your child.

Every parent is busy; parents of children with epilepsy may be even busier than most. This book has been organized with the busy parent in mind. The first four chapters are a "must read" for every parent. They provide the basic tools for understanding epilepsy, behavior management, and school programming. The final chapter summarizes parenting of a child with epilepsy in three key terms, providing an easy to remember checklist. The remainder of the book is organized so that you can turn to a section when you need it. Issues for parenting a toddler with epilepsy are far different from issues for parenting an adolescent. You can go to the information that you need, when you need it, returning to the book for an update as your child grows and new issues emerge. You can select the section that is important to you in understanding your child, then read the other chapters when you have time or want to know more about the brain in general.

Childhood epilepsy may provide speed-bumps in the road to adulthood, but it does not have to be a barricade. For 20 years, I have helped parents negotiate the speed bumps, creating an owner's manual for their child. Now, let me help you make this journey.

The Basic Tools

CHAPTER 1

Understanding Epilepsy

To understand epilepsy, you first need to understand how the brain works. The brain is composed of nerve cells. These cells generate tiny electrical discharges to get information from one end of the cell to the other. The electrical discharges cause the cell to release chemicals called *neurotransmitters* that carry the cell's message across the gap between cells. Some neurotransmitters tell the cell to fire, while others tell the cell to be quiet. For most people, this process proceeds in an orderly fashion. The tiny electrical discharges are organized, allowing us to do everything from running a race or learning new information to breathing and sleeping. Just like other brain activity, a *seizure* involves a burst of electrical activity. It may involve just a small cluster of cells (focal discharge) or the whole brain (generalized discharge). Seizures disrupt meaningful activity because the electrical pattern is abnormal. The abnormal pattern can result in the loss of consciousness, produce feelings unrelated to what is going on around the person, or produce movements that have no purpose.

If you have a brain, it is possible for you to have a seizure. Many things can cause a seizure to occur. Seizures can occur as part of an immediate medical problem. For example, in young children, a high fever can cause a seizure. Chemical imbalances in the body, such as low blood sugar, can cause a seizure. Infections involving the brain can cause a seizure. A sharp blow to the head can cause a seizure. Seizures are classified as *provoked* when there is an acute medical cause; that is, something is happening right now and that cause can be treated.

A seizure is classified as *unprovoked* where there is no acute medical cause. Epilepsy is diagnosed when a person has more than one unprovoked seizure.

▶ What causes epilepsy?

Some epilepsy is *symptomatic*, which means that the neurologist has identified a cause for the repeated seizures. Unlike a provoked seizure, the seizures in symptomatic epilepsy are the result of a chronic medical condition. For example, seizures may result from scar tissue that has formed in the brain. Scar tissue can result from an infection, a period of time when the brain is deprived of oxygen, a very high fever, or an injury to the brain resulting from an accident or stroke.

Small clusters of cells may fail to organize normally during development and become the source of seizures. Your doctor may refer to these clusters of cells as *cortical dysplasia* (malformed structure) or a *migrational disorder* (normal cells in an abnormal location). Although the first symptoms of most brain tumors in children are typically headaches or a change in coordination, seizures may be the first symptom of a brain tumor for some children. A brain imaging study, such as a magnetic resonance imaging (MRI) scan, is used to look for scars, tumors, cortical dysplasia, and migrational disorders when children initially develop seizures.

In recent years, research has discovered that some seizure disorders are genetic; that is, the tendency to have a certain type of seizure runs in the family. These genetic seizure syndromes typically respond well to medication. For some of the syndromes, the epilepsy is time-limited, and the child will eventually "outgrow" his seizures. Other genetic syndromes that involve the nervous system are associated with an increased risk of epilepsy. In other words, only some children with the syndrome will develop seizures. In disorders such as tuberous sclerosis or neurofibromatosis, seizures are often more difficult to control, and the child is less likely to outgrow them. Your physician will ask questions about your family's history of neurologic problems in looking for possible genetic causes for your child's epilepsy.

Although researchers are learning more about the causes of epilepsy, for most children with seizures the neurologist will not be able to identify a cause for the epilepsy. When a cause cannot be found, the seizures are referred to as ideopathic or cryptogenic.

▶ Do all seizures look the same?

There are many different types of seizures. A classification system was developed by the International League Against Epilepsy (ILAE) for physicians to use in describing seizures. The classification system divides seizures into two large classes: generalized seizures and partial seizures. For *generalized seizures,* the abnormal electrical activity involves the entire brain. As a result, the person having a generalized seizure loses consciousness during the seizure. In *partial seizures*, the abnormal electrical activity begins in a small portion of the brain, but can spread to involve the whole brain. During partial seizures, the person may remain aware to some degree, but may be confused or limited in her ability to respond to others.

When people think of seizures, most think of a *generalized tonic clonic seizure*, previously known as a *grand mal seizure*. The person experiencing the seizure slumps to the ground, is unconscious, and jerks his arms and legs. Other types of generalized seizures exist. Absence epilepsy, previously known as *petit mal seizures*, involves only a loss of consciousness. The child having absence spells may blink his eyes or stare off, with no other indication that the seizure is occurring. *Absence seizures* tend to be brief. Unless directly working with the child at the time of the seizure, a teacher or parent may not be aware that it occurred. Children with *myoclonic epilepsy* may have sudden jerks of the arms, shoulders, or head. *Tonic seizures* are characterized by an increase in muscle tone. During a tonic seizure, the child's body appears stiff, with arms and legs extended. An *atonic seizure* involves a sudden loss of muscle tone. During an atonic seizure, the child suddenly goes limp. Both tonic and atonic seizures can cause the child to fall without warning, and these sudden falls can result in injury to the child.

Partial seizures start in a small area of the brain. Think about all the different things that you can do, such as the ways you move and the sensations you experience. Depending on where seizures start, partial seizures can mimic many of the movements or feelings that are part of everyday life.

Simple partial seizures involve a sudden sensation that is not related to anything going on around the person. For example, if a simple partial seizure starts in parts of the brain responsible for interpreting what we see, the seizure may involve seeing colors or a pattern. If the seizure starts in the part of the brain responsible for emotions, the seizure may involve a sense of fear. Some simple partial seizures create a feeling of "butterflies" in the stomach or nausea. Prickly or tingling feelings in some part of the body, like when your foot has fallen asleep, may occur when simple partial seizures start in the part of the brain that interprets touch sensations. During simple partial seizures, the person remains aware of what is going on around him.

Complex partial seizures often involve movements that look purposeful. However, the actions are repeated over and over without accomplishing anything. For example, the person may smack her lips or pick at clothing. She may experience jerking or stiffening of a hand or leg. Since only a small part of the brain is involved, the person experiencing a partial seizure may still be able to hear what is being said or may be able to talk. However, awareness is reduced—the person may be confused or may hear but be unable to respond. Partial seizures may spread to other parts of the brain and even involve the whole brain. When this occurs, the seizure is described as *secondarily generalized.*

▶ **Are seizure types the same as seizure syndromes?**

A *seizure type* is a description of the behavior seen during the seizure and of the pattern of brain activity that occurs during the seizure. The classification system just described refers to seizure types. A *seizure syndrome* is a description of a group of symptoms that go together. The symptoms that define the syndrome include one or more seizure types as well as information about age of seizure onset, the likelihood that medication will control the seizures, and the likely effect the seizures will have on the child's development of cognitive skills. Every child with epilepsy has at least one seizure type but may not fit into a seizure syndrome.

▶ **How is epilepsy diagnosed?**

For some children, seizures become recognized through a medical emergency. The child has a generalized tonic clonic seizure or a prolonged complex partial seizure, parents or teachers know that something is wrong, and the child is taken to the emergency room. However, since seizures can mimic behaviors that children show every day, such as daydreaming, seizures may occur for a long time before anyone suspects that there is something wrong. Parents may even discuss concerns about their child's behavior with a physician and be told that it is "normal" or "just a phase." When these seizures are eventually diagnosed, parents may feel guilty for not knowing what was really wrong, or may become angry at the physician who didn't take their concerns seriously. While these are normal feelings, it is important for parents to focus on what they can do now for their child, not what they wished they had done in the past.

Physicians rely on descriptions of behavior from parents and other caregivers as the first step in making the diagnosis of epilepsy. The physician will want to know what you see your child doing that has you concerned, when the events happen, and what happens at the end of the event. At this point, your physician may refer you and your child to a pediatric neurologist for further medical evaluation.

The next step in the diagnosis of epilepsy is an *electroencephalogram* (EEG). For this test, small electrodes that look like little buttons are glued to the scalp (yes, the glue comes off). The neurologist may ask you to limit the amount of sleep that your child has before the test so that she will fall asleep during the test (sleep-deprived EEG). Some electrical abnormalities associated with seizures occur during sleep or as the child moves between sleep and wakefulness. Sleep depriving a child means that at least one parent has also been sleep deprived. If at all possible, a parent, relative, or friend who has gotten a full night's sleep should do the driving to keep the appointment for this sleep-deprived study. The results of the EEG will help the physician to determine what type of seizure your child is having and may provide information regarding the parts of the brain responsible for the seizure. The EEG, paired with your description of the seizures will help your physician to select the most appropriate type of medication for your child.

The neurologist may order a brain imaging study that provides a picture of brain structure. The neurologist is looking for changes in brain structure that might be a cause for the seizures. Most often, this will be a *magnetic resonance image* (MRI), a picture obtained through the use of magnetic fields rather than with x-rays. However, if your child's first seizure is treated in an emergency room, a *computerized tomography* (CT) scan (brain picture obtained with x-rays) may be obtained. A CT scan takes less time and is more readily available in an emergency setting. The pictures resulting from the CT scan do not have as much detail as the MRI scan. As a result, if your child has a CT scan, the physician may recommend that you get an MRI scan at a later date.

If the neurologist suspects that the seizures are the result of some other medical problem, blood tests or other laboratory studies may be conducted to help diagnose the syndrome.

▶ **How do I prepare my child for an EEG**
   and a brain imaging study?
What you do to prepare your child depends on her age. Preschool and elementary age children need to know what they will experience, while older children will need to know both "what" and "why." In explaining the EEG procedure, your child needs to know that buttons—the electrodes—will be put on her head with paste. The EEG technician may use what looks like a needle to put jelly in the electrodes. The child should be reassured that the EEG technician will not be giving her a shot. When the jelly is put in the electrodes, the child may feel a little scratch, as when she scratches her head with her fingernails. Getting ready for the EEG takes 20 to 30 minutes with a cooperative child.

During the procedure, your child will be asked to sit very still, to look at lights, and to breathe fast like she does when she has just finished running. She may be asked to close her eyes and try to fall asleep. A routine EEG lasts for about 40 minutes, while a sleep-deprived EEG lasts about an hour. When it is done, the EEG technician will remove the electrodes. The technician uses "smelly stuff " to get them off and will rub your child's head to get as much of the paste off as possible. Some children like to hold a towel over their nose so that they don't have to smell the paste remover.

You will want to wash your child's hair after the EEG. Parents have found that using conditioner, styling gel, or mousse helps to make the hair slippery, making it easier to get all of the paste to come off.

For an MRI scan, your child will be asked to lay very still on a long narrow table. The table will move into a tunnel (the magnet). The child may be given an IV so that *contrast material,* a dye, can be injected for some of the pictures. Depending on the type of pictures that your physician wants, MRI scans can take from 45 minutes to an hour.

Children who are too young to lie still or have difficulty lying still may be given sedation prior to the scan so that they will "sleep" while the scan is being done. If this is necessary, tell your child that she is coming to the hospital to get a picture taken of her brain, that some "sleepy medicine" will be needed to have the picture taken, and that you will be there and will take her home when the procedure is done.

For scans done without sedation, the first step may involve having an IV started. This will allow the MRI technician to inject some contrast material to get better pictures of the brain. Your child needs to know that this IV involves a needle going into the arm or hand, and that a little soft tube will stay in his blood vessel during the MRI. The tube will be taken out when the pictures are all done. Let the child know that it may hurt a little when the technician is putting the tiny tube in his arm, but that it will not hurt once the tube is placed. Next, the child will be asked to lie on the narrow table. The MRI technician will put pads on either side of his head, as well as using a head frame that comes over the front of the head, but does not cover up the face. You can describe this as being like a "space helmet." Straps may be used across the chest and legs to help the child remember to lie still. You can describe these to him as being like a "seatbelt" in the car. When the scanner is taking pictures the "engine" running the scanner will make noise. Most hospitals have earphones for the child to wear in the scanner so that he can listen to music during the scan, and some play a video tape during the scan. Your child will have a push-button to hold, to use if he needs help. Remind your child that he will need to stay very still so that the pictures do not turn out blurry.

▶ How is epilepsy treated?

Medications called *antiepileptic drugs* (AEDs) are most often used to treat epilepsy. For many children, a single AED will be effective in controlling seizures. However, for some children, seizures prove difficult to control and a combination of AEDs may be used. Your physician will start your child on a low dose of the AED, gradually increasing the dose over a series of days or weeks. This is so that the child's body can become used to the medication. The child will need to get blood tests so that the physician can tell how much of the medicine is in the blood stream, making it available to the brain. Blood tests may be frequent at the beginning of treatment, but less frequent as the seizures are controlled.

Any medication can have *side effects*. A side effect is something that the medication does in addition to treating the seizures. When we think of side effects, we typically are talking about an undesirable effect of the medicine. For AEDs, the most common side effects include sleepiness and tremor (shakiness). Some AEDs may affect behavior, with a child becoming more active or more moody and irritable. AEDs can also affect appetite. Your physician will provide you with information about common side effects when a medication is started. Some neurologists have Fact Sheets for each AED that summarize this information.

Not all children with epilepsy need to take medication to control their seizures. There are some syndromes in which seizures only occur during the night or as the child is waking up in the morning. In these cases, the side effects that may be associated with medication are felt to be more disruptive to the child than an occasional seizure.

▶ Will my child's seizures be controlled by medication?

Researchers have looked for ways to predict which children will have their seizures easily controlled with medication and those who will continue to have seizures. A recent study by Dr. A.T. Berg and her colleagues involving more than 600 children with newly diagnosed epilepsy found that seizures were controlled for 90% of the children. Very frequent seizures at the time of diagnosis and the presence of a known cause for the epilepsy lowered the odds that seizures would be controlled. Children with no known cause for their seizures had better odds that seizures would be controlled.

Research can give you a general sense of what happens to a group of children, but it does not tell you what will happen with *your* child. Your neurologist may be able to tell you how likely it is that your child's seizures will be controlled with medication. However, you should be prepared for the fact that the neurologist may only be able to suggest that you "wait and see."

▶ **What if medication does not work for my child?**
For some children, even combinations of AEDs are not effective in producing seizure control. When this occurs, your neurologist may talk to you about other approaches to treatment such as the ketogenic diet, neurosurgery to remove the seizure *focus* (its point of origin), or surgery to implant a vagal nerve stimulator.

The ketogenic diet is a very high fat diet that must be strictly followed to help the child. This means that she cannot eat the treats other children bring to school for special days. Often this means that the family prepare separate meals for the child. While this diet requires a major commitment from the family and child, families have found it to be worthwhile when it results in improvement in seizure control. To find out more about the ketogenic diet, you can talk with your neurologist or consult *The Ketogenic Diet: A Treatment for Epilepsy* by John Freeman, M.D. and colleagues.

The vagal nerve stimulator is a device much like a pacemaker. It is installed under the skin in the chest wall, with wires that wrap around the vagal nerve. The stimulator sends electrical impulses to the vagal nerve; the vagal nerve then sends these impulses on to the brain. The simulator is programmed by the neurologist to send electrical impulses at regular intervals. The child or parent has a magnet that he can touch to the child's skin over the stimulator to trigger these impulses. Children who can feel their seizures starting can trigger the stimulator to interrupt the seizures. While few children have had seizures totally controlled by this device, it has helped to reduce the frequency or severity of seizures for some children.

Surgery may be an option for children whose seizures start in only one part of the brain. Currently, children are considered for surgery only if more than one medication has been tried and has failed to control their seizures. If your child is felt to be a surgical candidate, your neurologist will most likely refer you to an epilepsy center that specializes in surgical evaluations.

The medical evaluation for surgery typically begins with a Video EEG. For this procedure, electrodes are placed as they would be for a routine EEG. Your child's head will be wrapped with gauze to keep the electrodes in place for one or more days of EEG recording. The EEG wires plug into a small box that the child can carry in a fanny pack or backpack. Your child will stay in a hospital room that contains a video camera and a hook-up for a cable to connect the electrode box to the recording equipment, and will be encouraged to go about his everyday activities. You will be with your child and will have a button to press whenever you observe seizures to be occurring. This allows the neurologist to detect behavior changes and correlate them with EEG changes. It helps the neurologist to determine whether seizures are coming from a single focus or from many areas of the brain.

As part of a surgical evaluation, your child may need to undergo *neuropsychological assessment*. Learning activities and "games" are presented that measure your child's development of many different types of skills such as language; drawing; interpreting sounds, visual information, or touch; memory; and organizational skills. School-related skills such as reading, math, and spelling, as well as general reasoning skills (IQ) are also assessed. Your child's pattern of strong skills and weak skills may help the neurologist to determine the area in the brain that is producing seizures. The results of testing are used to define the child's skills prior to surgery—to establish a skills baseline. Repeat testing is conducted following surgery. Results from post-surgical testing will be compared to presurgical testing to determine if changes in skills have occurred.

Additional brain imaging studies may be obtained during a surgical evaluation. Your child may have an MRI scan to provide more detailed pictures of brain structure in areas that are suspected to be producing the seizures. A *functional MRI* (fMRI) may be used to get information about brain areas involved in the performance of important skills such as movement or language. During a functional MRI, the child will be asked to perform a skill (e.g., move a finger, think of words) and the brain areas involved in performing this skill will be evident on the scan. Studies of brain activity (PET scan, SPECT scan) may be conducted during and between seizures to determine if your child has a single seizure focus and the location of that focus.

▶ **Who will help me with my child?**

When your child has epilepsy, you take on new responsibilities. However, you are not alone. Your physician and the nurses in your physician's office will be your first and most important source of information regarding the seizure disorder. Since there are many different seizure types and seizure syndromes, these medical personnel can guide you to information related to your child's specific situation.

The type of physician who helps you depends on your child's needs, the resources in your area, and your insurance plan. Your family physician or pediatrician may diagnose the epilepsy and start treatment. If your child's seizures are controlled, and he is not experiencing any problems, this physician can continue to care for him.

If seizures are not controlled, or if unacceptable side effects occur, your child is likely to be referred to a neurologist. In rural areas, this may be a neurologist who treats both children and adults. In urban areas, the neurologist who sees your child is likely to specialize in children (pediatric neurologist). The neurologist may take over your child's care, or may work with your local physician in managing her epilepsy.

If seizures continue to be difficult to control, the neurologist may refer you to a pediatric epileptologist. This is a neurologist who specializes in the treatment of childhood epilepsy. A pediatric epileptologist typically works in a comprehensive epilepsy program associated with a large hospital or medical school. If you live near a comprehensive epilepsy program, the pediatric epileptologist may take over your child's care. If you are traveling to see the epileptologist, she will work with a local physician in caring for your child.

Your physician may refer you to a psychologist or neuropsychologist to address concerns about your child's behavior and style of learning. The psychologist or neuropsychologist can work with you so that special learning needs can be addressed by your child's school. The psychologist or neuropsychologist will help you know what is appropriate to expect from your child and what to do if behavior problems occur. While psychologists are found in most areas, you may need to travel to a large city to work with a neuropsychologist.

▶ **Where can I turn to learn more about epilepsy?**

The Epilepsy Foundation has information for you, your family, and your child's school. You can contact the foundation by phone at 1-800-332-1000 or through the Internet at www.epilepsyfoundation.org. In addition to the national office, regional offices of the Epilepsy Foundation are located throughout the country. You can check your phone book to see if there is an office listed in your area, or you can get this information from the national office or its Web site.

To learn more about the diagnosis and medical treatment of epilepsy, consult *Seizures and Epilepsy in Childhood: A Guide for Parents* by Freeman, Vining, and Pilias.

If you enter the word "epilepsy" into an Internet search engine, you will find more than 100 sites. Be careful about the Internet sites that you visit. Epilepsy refers to many different seizure types and can be associated with many different medical conditions. Any given "epilepsy site" may not have information related to your child's seizures or seizure syndrome. Sites that are run by universities or by regional epilepsy centers (usually affiliated with medical schools or large hospitals) can be a good source of balanced, accurate information.

Web pages offering information on a single approach to treatment may not provide objective information about that approach or about treatment alternatives. Keep in mind that epilepsy in children is different from epilepsy in adults. If you see phrases such as "research suggests . . ." you need to know if the research involved children or adults. If it involved children, you need to know if the children had the same type of seizures as your child.

RECOMMENDED READING:

Freeman J, Freeman J, Kelly M. *The Ketogenic Diet Book: A Treatment for Epilepsy, 3rd Edition.* New York: Demos Medical Publishing, 2000.

Freeman JM, Vining EPG, Pillas D. Seizures and Epilepsy in Childhood: A Guide for Parents, 2nd Edition. Baltimore: The Johns Hopkins University Press, 1997.

CHAPTER 2

The Challenges of Living with Epilepsy

▶ **Will I be able to predict when seizures will occur?**
Children vary greatly in the frequency with which they experience seizures. Some children have seizures many times a day while others may have only one or two a year. For some children, seizures are totally controlled with medication after the first few seizures that resulted in the diagnosis of epilepsy and treatment with medication. For other children, seizures continue, but may be less frequent or shorter than they were prior to treatment. Seizure frequency may fluctuate, with the child having "good days" and "bad days."

Some children have a pattern to their seizures. If a seizure is going to occur, it tends to occur at the same time of day. For example, for some seizure syndromes, seizures occur when the child is tired or as he is falling asleep or waking up. Seizures starting in the frontal lobes of the brain have a tendency to occur during sleep.

For some children, seizures appear to be related to certain activities. Some seizures are triggered by patterns of light. These are called photo-sensitive seizures. During a routine EEG, the technician uses a flashing light to check for this type of seizure. For some children, exercise or heat appears to trigger seizures. Although uncommon, a few children present with *reflex epilepsy*, in which a specific activity, such as reading, triggers a seizure.

Some children experience an *aura* right before a seizure. An aura is a sensation that actually signals the beginning of the seizure. When a child experiences an aura, she may have enough time to come to you or to let someone else know that a seizure is about to occur.

For many children, seizures occur without a predictable pattern or without a warning. Because you would like to be prepared to help your child, it is tempting to look for a pattern even when none exists. For example, if your child has a seizure right after you have firmly told him to pick up his toys, you may conclude that being firm with your child causes seizures. It is easy to remember the times that discipline was followed by a seizure and to forget the times that seizures occurred when your child was enjoying an activity.

The best way to determine if your child's seizures follow a predictable pattern or have a "trigger" is to keep a *seizure calendar*. A seizure calendar is a record of each seizure that your child has over a series of weeks or months (depending on seizure frequency). The seizure calendar does not have to include extensive description of each seizure. You can make a list of your child's seizure types if she demonstrates seizures in more than one way. For the calendar you simply record day, time of day, what the child was doing immediately before the seizure, and the seizure type (see Table 2.1). You can review this record with your neurologist to see if a pattern emerges.

TABLE 2.1

Sample Seizure Calendar

Seizure Code:

Type 1: Stares, picks at clothing with left hand, understands what is said,but can't respond

Type 2: Stares, unresponsive

Type 3: Funny feeling in the tummy

DATE	TIME	TYPE	ACTIVITY AT TIME OF SEIZURE	ACTIVITY FOLLOWING SEIZURE
5/2	12:30 PM	2	Eating lunch	Continued eating; no prompt from parent needed
5/9	3:45 PM	1	Doing homework	Rested for 15 minutes. Needed help remembering the task
5/14	3:30 PM	3, then 1	Told to pick up toys	Complained of being too tired to pick up toys. Watched TV until supper.
5/22	4:30 PM	1	Playing video game	Rested for 15 minutes. Restarted game.

▶ **Can my family still pursue activities that we enjoy?**

Family life does not come to a stop because your child has been diagnosed with epilepsy. Your family will not be the same as it was before your child's diagnosis. Some things will change in your family's day-to-day life due to your child's seizures and the medication needed to treat them. However, you can still do most things that your family enjoyed doing before the seizures. The fact that your child has seizures may require you to do more planning for some of these activities. If an activity has been important to your family in the past or is part of a family tradition, don't assume that you will no longer be able to do it. Talk with your neurologist to help identify a way to make the activity safe.

For example, if you enjoy wilderness camping and your child experiences prolonged seizures, you may want to talk with your neurologist about medication that you can take with you to treat these seizures. You may want to invest in a cell phone and make sure that your camping remains in areas where you can use the phone to get medical assistance if it became necessary. You might want to camp in a park near an urban area rather than in a wilderness preserve, a compromise that allows you to enjoy nature while still being near medical care.

Seizures themselves are seldom a threat to family activities, but the financial expenses related to the treatment of epilepsy may limit the amount of money that is left for family activities. If this happens, view it as an opportunity to try new things. You can do many inexpensive things as a family. Create adventures. A picnic in the park can be a treat to a child who has not done that before. A nature hike around the neighborhood can turn a regular walk into a special learning adventure. Create new family traditions. Many families rediscovered the joy of reading with their children each night while sharing the Harry Potter series. Children love to help in the kitchen, and an afternoon together making cookies may be as much of a treat to them as a trip to the movies. Children value some individual time with Mom or Dad every bit as much as they value material possessions.

Many families today are faced with juggling work schedules, each child's extracurricular activities, and each child's homework needs. For most families, being organized is the key to balancing these needs. When you have a child with epilepsy, you have a few more things to fit into that balance. Medical routines and doctor's appointments can divert parent's time and attention from other family activities. When learning problems accompany epilepsy, helping your child complete homework may leave less time for other family members. You may find that you have to plan "dates" with your spouse and each child in the family to ensure that everyone's needs, including your own, are getting met.

▶ **Will my child still be able to do the things that she enjoys?**
Tell your neurologist what your child enjoys and ask if she can continue these activities. The International League Against Epilepsy (ILEA) has published general guidelines, and your neurologist can help you apply these to your child. In determining the appropriateness of activities for your child, you and your neurologist must consider the specific characteristics of your child, characteristics of her seizure disorder, and characteristics of the activity. The goal is to maximize the child's options while minimizing the risk for serious injury.

In considering the characteristics of your child, think about things that would be considered by any parent in selecting activities for a child. Age is an important variable. With increasing age, children develop the physical skills (balance and coordination) and cognitive skills (attention, memory, imagination, judgment) that allow for successful participation in activities. If your child has physical limitations or is developing cognitive skills at a slower pace than other children, activities appropriate for most children of the same chronologic age may not be a good choice.

Some restrictions are related to seizure type. If seizures result in a loss of consciousness, you would not want your child to go hang gliding, scuba diving, rock climbing, or dangle from the top of the monkey bars. Seizures that affect control in an arm and hand, even if your child remains conscious, would also make these activities dangerous. However, it is important to consider the time of day when seizures occur in making decisions about these activities, some of which may be acceptable for children whose seizures only occur during sleep or at the time of awakening.

Some restrictions are related to activities that trigger seizures. Children whose seizures are sensitive to light patterns may not be able to play some or all video games. Children whose seizures are triggered by physical exertion may not be able to go out for track, but may be able to play golf.

Some restrictions make good sense for everyone. No one should swim alone. Everyone is safer swimming in a pool than in a lake or ocean. Everyone should wear a helmet when riding a bike, using roller blades, or riding a skateboard. These "restrictions" are things that make good sense for all children and for their parents too.

If you have a teenager, one limit is defined by law: Your teenager will not be allowed to drive if he has seizures. States differ in the length of time for which an individual must have seizure control in order to get a driver's license. Appendix B summarizes driving regulations by state.

Most children with seizures can still participate in sports, enjoy time with friends, and do the things that everyone else their age does. Your child can have chores and be expected to help out around the house. Your child can go to school and learn. As with family activities, your child's participation in the things she enjoys or is expected to do may just take a little more planning.

▶ **What will other people think?**

Unfortunately, epilepsy continues to be misunderstood. *Myths* are stories that have no basis in fact, *misconceptions* are ideas accepted as fact, and *stereotypes* are information that may be true for a limited number of people in a group, but that are not true of everyone. Myths, misconceptions, and stereotypes regarding epilepsy are common. How someone reacts to the information that your child has epilepsy will be related to the accuracy of the information that person has about epilepsy. Your job is to provide accurate information.

First, you need to get accurate information yourself. Your neurologist may have pamphlets to get you started, and the Epilepsy Foundation has pamphlets that you can share. Second, you need to be a good role model. If you continue to treat your child as a capable, responsible person, others will follow your lead and view your child in the same light. If you treat your child as "sick" or "fragile," others will do the same.

▶ **Whom do I tell?**

The answer to this question depends somewhat on your child's age. This question is addressed in more detail in the age-specific chapters that follow. First, you need to tell your family, including extended family members (siblings, grandparents, aunts, uncles, cousins). Trying to keep epilepsy a secret within the family is like trying to ignore an elephant in the living room—it can be done, but it is a lot of work. By trying to keep it a secret, it tells your child that he has a disease that is so horrible that no one can talk about it. Obviously, this may do bad things to your child's self-esteem. Telling family members is a good place to practice what you are going to say to others. It will help you find out what questions are likely to be asked and allow you to get more information before you take on people outside the family.

Second, you need to tell any adult who may be responsible for your child if she has a seizure. This may include school staff, coaches, and the parents of your child's friends. You want them to feel calm and in control if a seizure occurs. You want them to know what to do—and what not to do—for your child during and after a seizure.

Third, you may need to help your child tell his friends in an age appropriate fashion. In the age-specific chapters that follow, suggestions are provided for informing your child's friends in a manner appropriate to each developmental level.

If your child's seizure occur only during sleep or if they are controlled by medication, you may not need to tell as many people as you would if your child was experiencing intermittent seizures during the day. However, responsible adults in your child's life (including peers during the teen-age years) need to know that your child is on medication. If a medical emergency should occur, the treating physician needs this information. Some families choose to have their child wear a medic alert bracelet to address this need.

▶ **Does epilepsy make my child handicapped?**

A *handicap* is defined as something that hinders a person, placing him at a disadvantage. Having epilepsy does not make your child handicapped. However, it can have a serious effect on your child's feelings about himself. Research by Dr. Joan Austin and her associates have looked at the effect of a diagnosis of epilepsy on self-esteem, by comparing children with epilepsy to children with asthma. Asthma was chosen because, like epilepsy, it is a chronic medical condition that involves daily medication and regular doctor visits, and it can result in unpredictable "attacks." She found that ratings of self-esteem were significantly lower for those with epilepsy than for the children with asthma. The incidence of depression and behavior problems was higher in the group of children with epilepsy than in the asthma group. *This does not have to happen.* You can help your child develop and maintain positive self-esteem and age-appropriate behavior. You can make sure that your child remains an active, important member of your family.

It is important to recognize that the diagnosis of epilepsy has not made your child a different person from who he was before the diagnosis. It has just provided you with additional information about your child. He still needs praise, hugs, and kisses. He still needs discipline. If you have concerns regarding what is fair to expect, a psychologist or neuropsychologist can help you to identify your child's strengths and weaknesses, then help you to set expectations that build on the strengths and compensate for the weaknesses.

It is important to maximize the "normal" life experiences for your child. A study by Dr. Jane Williams found that children with epilepsy were more likely to sleep with their parents than were children with other chronic health conditions. If your child did not sleep with you before the diagnosis, you do not need to invite her into the bedroom after the diagnosis. If seizures occur at night, a nursery monitor in your child's room allows independence while still providing you with a means for knowing if she is having a seizure. If your child was bathing alone prior to the diagnosis of seizures, she should still have privacy in the bathroom once seizures are diagnosed. However, if your child loses consciousness during seizures, you will want her to take a shower rather than a bath and make sure that the bathroom door remains unlocked. Some parents have placed a nursery monitor in the bathroom to allow their teenager to have privacy while showering, yet allow parents to know if a seizure occurs.

▶ **How will this change our family?**
While the goal is to keep your family life as "normal" as possible, having a child with epilepsy does mean that parents take on new roles. You may become a "nurse" in that you need to administer medications each day. You may become a "physician's assistant," keeping seizure records and behavioral descriptions for the neurologist. You will become an "epilepsy educator," helping others to accurately understand your child's seizure disorder. You may become a "patient advocate" or "accountant," dealing with your insurance company and tracking your child's bills. You may become an "educational advocate," making sure that your child's school program is appropriate to his needs. Each of these potential roles takes some time.

Brothers and sisters may need to take on the role of "helper" during seizures. Because parents are busy with their new roles, all children in the family may have new chores so that there can be time left for family fun.

Brothers and sisters may initially be angry about changes in family life. They may become jealous of the time you spend with the child with seizures, or of the attention he now gets from others. It is important to have a little private time with each child in your family. Going for a walk together or spending a few minutes alone together prior to tucking the child in for the night can provide opportunities for siblings to share their feelings. Teachers, parents of friends, or relatives may also be good sources of information regarding how siblings are feeling.

Sometimes when a child is diagnosed with epilepsy, relatives become more involved in the family. Grandparents, aunts, and uncles may decide to become an epilepsy information source, searching the Internet for treatment suggestions. Friends and neighbors may share suggestions about what worked for someone else's child. This assistance can be a good thing or a bad thing.

It is a good thing when information is offered as an "option" for you to think about or discuss with your neurologist. It is a bad thing when the relative or friend attempts to direct your child's care. You need to set limits, making it clear that *you* will make the final decisions regarding your child's treatment.

▶ **What impact will my child's epilepsy have on my relationship with my spouse?**

When a child experiences any chronic medical condition, it puts additional stress on the parents' relationship with each other. As your lives become busier, it is important that you find time for one another. It is important that you have time to share information about *all* your children. It is important that you have time to discuss expectations for each child, to set consistent household rules, and to agree on consequences for rule violation. It is important that you have time to talk openly about finances and budgeting.

Often one parent becomes responsible for taking the child to medical appointments. However, both parents need information from the treatment team to understand their child's needs and to make good decisions for her. Prior to medical appointments, it can help to make a list of questions that will be asked. The parent attending can take the list along and write down answers. Some physicians may be willing to take calls from the parent who cannot attend the appointment or schedule a separate time to meet with both parents together if a major decision needs to be made.

Sometimes children with epilepsy have parents who are divorced. Sometimes these parents have remarried, adding step-parents to the caring network surrounding the child with epilepsy. Communication remains the key for helping your child. Your neurologist must be aware of custody arrangements, particularly whether one or both of you retain the right to make medical decisions. If one parent is not allowed access to medical information, your neurologist needs to know this as well. If both parents will make medical decisions, both need to have access to the neurologist to make sure that they understand the child's medical needs. When step-parents are involved, it helps for all parents to understand early in the child's treatment what role each caring adult will play in treatment decisions.

▶ **Is the impact of epilepsy on the family any different than the impact of other chronic childhood health problems?**

Epilepsy is no different than other chronic childhood medical conditions in that the diagnosis can mean changes in family roles and challenges to family finances. For any chronic medical condition, parents need a means of communicating with each other and with the treating physician. Epilepsy does differ from other medical conditions in that there is still a great deal of misunderstanding associated with this diagnosis. You will need to work harder to educate others so that your child's life remains as "normal" as possible.

CHAPTER 3

Dealing with the Demon
at the Dinner Table

J UST LIKE ANY CHILD, children with epilepsy misbehave. Unlike other children, parents and teachers often feel confused about how to respond to this misbehavior. What if it is a seizure? What if the medication is making him act that way? What if discipline makes her have a seizure? Too often, misbehavior is ignored as parents attempt to find the answers to these questions. Too often, ignoring misbehavior results in more misbehavior and in the child's learning socially inappropriate coping strategies.

▶ **Why do children misbehave?**
All children misbehave as they learn ways to cope. Coping behaviors include ways to express feelings, to protect themselves from negative experiences, and to balance their needs with other's needs. Providing a child with structure and limits provides a safety net as she explores means for coping. Failing to provide discipline and guidance into more socially acceptable ways of coping robs the child of this security and of an important learning experience.

Children misbehave to achieve a goal. The goal may be to rid themselves of an uncomfortable feeling such as frustration, anger, fear, or sadness. The goal may be to avoid frightening or frustrating situations. The goal may be to gain adult attention. The goal may be to demonstrate limited competence so that help is always available. The goal may be to test the limits to make sure that her safety net is dependable. When you understand the goal, you will understand how to help your child learn a more appropriate way to meet it.

▶ **Why is discipline important?**
Discipline is important for two reasons. First, it helps your child to learn

age-appropriate ways to cope with problems and resolve conflicts. This gives your child the opportunity to be successful as he leaves home, initially to play with others, then to go to school, and eventually to live on his own. Second, it provides your child with a sense of security. Emotional reactions can leave a child feeling overwhelmed and out of control. Consistent discipline lets your child know that you will not let his actions go too far. Your child will know that he is safe because you are there to help.

▶ **Why is it more difficult to apply this process to children with epilepsy?**
The presence of seizures and medication often cloud the process. Questions about possible seizure activity may be substituted for questions regarding the goal of the misbehavior. Questions involving effects of medications may interfere with action to help the child learn a more appropriate behavior. Parents frequently are immobilized with a sense that the child is a "victim" of seizures and medication. From there, parents conclude: "Maybe she couldn't help it." If the misbehavior has no goal, there is no need for discipline and the teaching that goes with it. At least, not until the parents are certain that she really meant to do it. If this level of certainty regarding intention is not reached, the family becomes hostage to a "demon at the dinner table."

▶ **How can I tell if my child is misbehaving or is having a seizure?**
If your child has seizures characterized by staring, this question may arise when she does not respond to the direction that you have just given. How can you be sure that you were heard and understood? You use the same approach as parents whose children do not have epilepsy use to make sure that they are understood.

- Reduce competition for your attention. If your child is watching TV, turn it off or stand between the child and the screen. If she is playing with toys, use your hands to interrupt the play, holding the child's hands.
- Use your child's name or touch her to make eye contact. Some parents have found it helpful to use a phrase such as "Give me your eyes" as a cue for their child to make eye contact with parents when expected to listen. If your child is looking at you, she is more likely to be listening to you.
- Give the direction in the form of a command, not a request. A request allows your child choice in complying ("Would you like to

get ready for bed?"). A command makes it clear that *you* are controlling the range of choices ("It is time to get ready for bed. Do you want to brush your teeth first or put on your pajamas?")

- While giving the command, watch your child's reaction. Look for signs of typical seizure. If you see seizure activity, re-orient the child and give the direction again.
- Have the child show you what he is expected to do. Many children can repeat back what they have heard, but still do not know how to turn that information into action. By having your child demonstrate what was commanded, you can be sure the child understood. Demonstration has the added bonus of getting your child started on the task.
- If you return to find your child is off-task, the reason for being off-task (seizure, distraction, didn't want to do it) makes no difference. Redirect the child to the task. You can either remain to supervise task completion or let her know that you will check back to make sure the task is done.

When children have complex partial seizures, questions may arise regarding whether or not aggressive behavior was the result of a seizure. Observing the kind of aggression that has occurred usually provides an answer to this question. Children experiencing complex partial seizures may react with aggressive behavior if someone attempts to restrain their movement. This reflects the fact that the child is confused. The aggression is in the form of combative behavior, attempting to get away from the restraint. Combative behavior will occur regardless of who provides the restraint. *Automatisms*, repetitive actions during a seizure, may inadvertently lead to destruction of papers on which the child is working or of material handled during the seizure. Children experiencing automatisms demonstrate the same type of automatism with each seizure, with damage to property only occurring if something happens to be within reach. During seizures, individuals do not become aggressive in the sense of seeking out and hurting others. When Joey slugs his sister or Suzie pinches her brother, this is not a seizure. During a seizure, it is unlikely that a child would go through a few rooms in the house, arrive in a sibling's room, and then break the sibling's new toy. If you are unsure about your child's aggressive actions, talk to your neurologist. She may be able to provide an answer or may recommend a prolonged EEG recording to capture the behavior that concerns you.

▶ **Should children with frequent seizures or associated attention problems be expected to complete tasks assigned to them?**

If the task is appropriate to your child's abilities, he should be expected to complete it. Children with frequent seizures or attention problems can be provided with a checklist that outlines the steps they are expected to complete. Involve your child in making the checklist by talking about each step for the task, and asking him to suggest a key word or phrase to remind him of the step. For young children, pictures can be substituted for the phrases or key words on the checklist. For frequently occurring tasks, such as daily chores, a wipe off board or laminated checklist allows your child to actually mark off each item as it is completed.

Initially the number of steps on the list should be kept small. You may need to check frequently to ensure that your child is making progress with the list. If the child is off-task, interrupt her and prompt her to look at the list, helping her to recognize what she should be doing. As your child learns to use the checklist, you will be able to gradually reduce the amount of supervision you provide.

▶ **What if the medication is making my child act this way?**

There are two types of medication side effects . First, changes in behavior can be the direct consequence of the medication. Medications differ in their likelihood of producing behavioral side effects and in the kind of side effects they produce. For example, phenobarbital may produce problems with impulsivity and hyperactivity in some children that are consistent with the condition Attention Deficit/Hyperactivity Disorder (ADHD). Other medications such as valproate (Depakote®) and topiramate (Topamax®) are associated with increased irritability in some children. For some medications, behavioral side effects are consistently related to use of the drug. For others, side effects may occur only at certain doses, or only as the child is getting used to the drug. Since children react differently to medications, it is important that you use experience with your own child rather than base your decision on what happened to some other child on this medication.

Medications may also have indirect effects on your child's emotional status. Indirect effects occur when side effects of a medication provide your child with a new challenge with which to cope. For example, medication may make your child more fatigued or increase his appetite. Introduction of a medication may make your child feel different, such as light-headed or dizzy. Skill changes, such as a fine tremor that slows writing speed, slowed thinking, or word finding problems, may increase his level of frustration. An increase in frustration during the school day may result in irritable or moody behavior when your child comes home. For young children, the lack of an effective vocabulary to talk about these changes may produce fear and confusion; these in turn may result in an increase in clingy behavior, irritability, and moodiness.

▶ **How can I tell if medication is responsible?**
You need to be a good observer, a good detective. Ask yourself the following questions:

- Is this a new behavior or the more frequent occurrence of a behavior that my child has occasionally demonstrated in the past?
- When did the behavior change occur? Is there a relationship between the behavior and a change in medication?
- Does the behavior occur all the time? Is there a pattern involving problems only at certain times of day? Is the behavior worse during the week or on the weekend?
- Does the behavior occur everywhere? Is it a problem at school? Have my child's friends noticed a change during playtime? Is it just a problem at home?
- What else is going on in my child's life? Keep in mind that children with epilepsy are not immune to the many other normal stresses encountered in childhood and adolescence. Childhood stresses include: moving to a new home; parent change in employment (going to work, new hours); death of a family member, friend, or pet; illness of family member; parental conflict, separation, divorce; natural disaster (tornadoes, hurricanes, floods); highly publicized criminal behavior (e.g., school shootings); and puberty.

▶ **Now that I have investigated, what do I do with the information I have gained?**
The key to understanding whether or not medication is playing a role is to look for timing. If medication is contributing to behavior change, you would expect to see the emergence of the behavior or an increase in its frequency after a medication change. Some behaviors are dose related, and occur when the medication is at its highest or lowest level in the blood stream. For dose-related effects, behavior problems tend to happen at the same time each day. Behaviors related to medication change are usually evident in more than one setting. If problems occur only in one setting, the behavior change is less likely to be medication related.

▶ **If medication is responsible, now what do I do?**

There are two answers to this question: change the medication or deal directly with the behavior.

You need to share your observations with your neurologist. Working together, you need to discuss the potential benefits of the medication and the potential problems that your child's behavior poses. Sometimes, the neurologist can suggest another medication that would be equally effective. The neurologist may ask you to give the current medication more time to see if behavior improves as your child adapts to it. In some cases, he may encourage you to work on managing the behavior because the medication seems to be the best option for controlling your child's seizures.

When the neurologist encourages you to manage the behavior, two approaches can be taken—you can try to contain the behavior, or you can work on teaching your child a different, more appropriate way to deal with the emotional or physical changes that resulted in the inappropriate behavior. *Containing* the behavior means that you accept that the behavior will occur and focus on changing the environment so that the behavior becomes a less serious problem. *Changing* behavior involves the teaching of new coping strategies. Let's explore each of these options.

Some medications make a child moody or irritable. The child appears to be on an emotional roller coaster. Often aggressive behavior, either verbal outbursts or evidence of physical aggression, occur with little to no warning. While the child's irritability is related to the medication, the child can be taught other ways of managing the expression of this feeling. The child is taught to change her coping strategy. For irritable behavior, the child can be taught to recognize when anger is increasing and to leave the situation before losing control (time away). Taking *time away* is a means of containing irritable or aggressive behavior. This approach works best when the child is helped to identify a means for releasing her feelings. In other words, the child is taught a new coping strategy. For example, she may be sent to her bedroom (time away) and encouraged to hit a pillow or rip up old newspapers (coping strategy). The child may be taught to take a few deep breaths and count to 10 (coping strategy). Family members and teachers can learn to "disengage," allowing the child the opportunity to regain control rather than getting into a power struggle with her. This intervention focuses on containing the problem by addressing an environmental factor that contributes to the inappropriate behavior.

While an approach involving interventions to both change and contain misbehavior is most often used, some skill changes related to medication can only be addressed through strategies to contain the medication's effects. Some medications may result in a skill change such as decreased impulse control, decreased attention span, difficulty retrieving words, tics, or tremor. For these types of problems, the environment must be changed to contain the problem, limiting the effects of the skill change on daily functioning. For impulsivity and hyperactivity, this may involve adding structure in the environment through increased supervision and more clearly defined rules and boundaries. The disruptive effects of tremor on handwriting can often be avoided by using computer technology as a means for completing written work. The effects of word finding problems on skill demonstration in school can be reduced by the use of recognition format tests (e.g., multiple choice, matching, true/false) rather than tests that involve the retrieval of facts learned (e.g., fill-in-the-blank, short answer, essay). When tics (involuntary, repetitive movements or vocalization) are present, it is important to educate teachers and friends so that the child is not punished or teased for the tics. See the Model Individual Education Plan in Appendix A for additional ways to contain medication effects.

▶ **What fears get in the way of effective consistent discipline for children with epilepsy?**

- *The "if I discipline my child, he will have a seizure" fear.* Many parents express fear that discipline will result in emotional upset, which in turn will trigger a seizure. While this is rarely the case, let's look at the reasoning that contributes to this thinking.

For most children, seizures are a random event. They can occur at any time, without warning. If a seizure occurs while the child is sleeping, few parents would conclude that they should not let the child sleep. If a seizure occurs while the child is engaged in an enjoyable activity such as going to a friend's birthday party, few parents would conclude that the child should never go to another birthday party. If a seizure occurs during an important activity, such as while attending reading class, few parents would conclude that the child should never learn to read. Some moments are part of life (sleeping), part of growing up (enjoying a party), or too important to be avoided (learning to read). However, some parents view discipline as something negative that they are expected to do *to* their child, rather than as a positive learning experience *for* their child. Thus, if discipline is associated with a seizure, discipline is optional. Discipline is put off, with the thought that they will discipline their child when seizures are controlled. After all, the reasoning goes, the child already has too much to cope with because she has seizures.

This line of thinking is faulty in two respects. First, children gain security from knowing that there are rules and boundaries. If the rules that they have trusted are suddenly changed, children experience more rather than less emotional distress. Relaxing the rules for one child also affects that child's relationships with others in the family or the classroom. Other children will rightly complain that "it isn't fair," becoming angry with the child with seizures and increasing stress for that child. Second, if the stress of discipline does "cause" a seizure, then it is important to help the child learn how to cope with this stress. Children learn coping strategies by facing the problem causing the stress, not by avoiding the stressful situation. Every child will experience negative consequences for behavior from someone. Every child needs to learn how to handle it. While parents feel that they are doing the child a favor by avoiding discipline, they are in fact making their child's life more difficult by their actions.

- *The "I don't know what is fair to expect of my child" fear.* This fear is most often expressed when children demonstrate fluctuations in important skills such as language comprehension or motor control related to seizures or medications. The parent gives a direction, the child fails to follow it, and the parent then begins to "second guess" whether the child understood what was said, or was currently incapable of following through. Out of concern for fairness, the parent decides to "let it go" and ignore the child's failure to follow through. While motivated by good intentions, the child will view the parent's actions as confusing and inconsistent. By trying to be fair and by attempting to make life easier for the child, the parent has acted in a manner that makes life more unpredictable, and therefore more difficult, for the child. What can a parent do?

First, *look at the relationship between the skill change and the command that was given or the rule that was broken.* For example, if a child's understanding of language fluctuates with seizures, the child still can be expected to follow well-learned household rules such as wearing a helmet when riding a bicycle or putting dirty clothes in the clothes hamper. When there is no relationship between the skill change and the command given or rule broken, the child deserves to experience the usual consequence of his misbehavior.

Second, *adapt commands to the child's current skill level.* For example, a child who experiences reduced control in one hand following seizures can still be expected to be dressed in time for school, but may not have to do all of the clothing fasteners independently. A child whose language comprehension declines after seizures can still be expected to pick up toys in response to a parent's command, but you may need to use a picture, gestures, or a demonstration to be certain that the child understands the command.

Third, *be consistent*. You may change the content of commands, the frequency with which you give commands, or the manner in which the command is given in response to skill changes following seizures. However, it is essential that when you give a command, you also enforce it.

Fourth, *some rules are too important to ever be broken*. It is never OK to intentionally throw and break your mother's table lamp. It is never OK to give your brother a bloody nose or bite your teacher. It is never OK to play in the middle of a busy street. If seizures are followed by increased irritability or impulsivity, your child will feel more secure knowing that you will increase your supervision to make sure that these behaviors do not happen, rather than "forgiving" him when they do.

▶ **Where can I turn for help?**
A number of books have been written for parents on behavior and discipline. You can start at your local library or check with your local school district. Some schools provide parenting groups through community education programs. The school psychologist, guidance counselor, or social worker may also be able to direct you to appropriate reading material. Representative books regarding discipline are listed at the end of the age-specific chapters that follow.

Seek professional help. A child psychologist or psychiatric social worker can work with you and your family in applying general parenting principles to the unique demands of your family and your resources. To find a good behavioral therapist, you can ask for recommendations from your child's neurologist, your family physician, or the social worker, psychologist, or counselor in your child's school.

CHAPTER 4

Epilepsy Goes to School

▶ **Should I tell the school that my child has epilepsy?**

If your child had diabetes or a heart condition, would you tell the school? Most people would say "Yes, of course." But heart conditions or diabetes do not carry the stigma that unfortunately remains associated with epilepsy. Parents fear that their child will be viewed as "brain damaged" or less capable of learning. Parents fear that other children with tease their child, or avoid her. Parents fear that telling the school will set in motion actions and events that will damage their child's self esteem. However, there are three good reasons for telling school personnel your child has epilepsy: reducing stigma, protecting self-esteem, and ensuring your child gets appropriate treatment in a medical emergency.

By not telling the school that your child has seizures, you may be contributing to stigma. School personnel will miss the opportunity to learn about the range of seizure manifestations, and fail to gain the personal experiences that provide the basis for understanding. They will have no reason to make epilepsy education a priority for themselves or for their students. Ignorance sustains stigma. Education and personal experience reduces stigma.

Your child knows that he has seizures. If you don't tell school personnel, you have to tell your child to keep this information a secret as well. Your child can't tell his teacher about this important thing in his life. He can't tell his friends because someone at school might find out. Your actions are telling your child that seizures are so bad that no one can find out about them. It is not surprising that such a message would have a negative impact on your child's feelings of worth (self-esteem).

If your child only has seizures during sleep and is not being treated with medication, you do not have to inform the school that your child has epilepsy. However, if your child is on medication, the school needs to know what medication he is taking even if you do not provide the reason why it is given. Although rare, emergencies can happen at school. Children fall and break a bone. Children sprain ankles. Children run into each other, knock heads, and briefly lose consciousness. If your child needs emergency medical care, you want school personnel to be able to provide all the information necessary to the emergency medical staff so that they can help him.

▶ **How do I deal with fear and ignorance?**

Don't assume that your school has accurate information about your child's epilepsy. Remember that epilepsy refers to recurrent unprovoked seizures, but that these seizures may take many different forms. For example, the school may have had a child who experienced epilepsy in the form of generalized tonic clonic seizures, and therefore might approach your child's absence seizures with the same interventions and restrictions. It is your job to provide the school with resources to help them get accurate information.

Contact the Epilepsy Foundation via the Internet at *www.epilepsyfoundation.org* or by phone at 1-800-332-1000. The Epilepsy Foundation is a wonderful source of written information for your school. It can also provide you with the name and location of the regional Epilepsy Foundation chapter closest to you. Some of the regional chapters have an educational team that can go to your child's school to provide an in-service workshop for school staff. Some of these chapters can also provide an in-service workshop for your child's class. Materials listed in the Foundation's on-line bookstore can be helpful in educating children with epilepsy, their peers, and their teachers. A catalog for this bookstore can be mailed to you if you do not have Internet access.

▶ **How do I prepare my child for questions from classmates?**

The answer to this question is related to your child's age. What is appropriate for helping the preschool- or kindergarten-age child would not be appropriate for the student in high school. Specific suggestions for helping your child talk with peers about her epilepsy are included in the age-specific chapters that follow.

In general, your child needs a label for her seizures. For young children, this label often reflects something about the child's experience during a seizure, while for older children and adolescents the label often is "seizure." In addition to having a label for the behavior that they might see, peers need to know what they should do to help during a seizure ("Get the teacher." "Just wait for it to stop.") Children need to practice what they will say to peers. For younger children, this can be accomplished through role playing (i.e., the parent pretends to be the child's friend). For older children and adolescents, the child may want to practice with a good friend before taking on other students.

▶ **What does the school need to know?**

School personnel need to have a current, accurate behavioral description of your child's seizures as well as the medical classification (generalized, complex partial, or other). This description should include what the teacher might see before a seizure. Some seizures have warnings, such as staring, repeatedly swallowing, a funny sensation, or seeing colored patterns. The teacher needs to know what will occur during the seizure and how long it will typically last. Will your child's eyes or head turn? Will he stop work and stare? Will he fumble with clothing? What will his hands, arms, and legs do? Finally, the teacher needs to know what happens when the seizure ends. Will your child be able to immediately return to work? Will he be confused? Will he need to sleep before being able to return to school activities? Will some aspect of your child's skills change after a seizure? If your child has more than one type of seizure, the school should be provided with this information for each type of seizure manifestation.

School personnel need to know what you do for your child during a seizure. Do they need to protect your child from falling or guide your child if she begins to wander? Should they just observe the seizure while providing reassurance to other students? Will they need to help your child get back on task when the seizure is over? Will your child need a change of clothes at school due to incontinence during the seizure?

They also need to know if you want to be informed of every seizure that occurs at school. If you want to be informed, do they need to call you as soon as a seizure occurs, or simply send home notes to let you know how many seizures were seen during the day? Do you want the school to keep a seizure log, sharing it with you on a weekly or monthly basis?

School personnel should be told when to consider your child's seizure a medical emergency. Are there specific types of seizures or a length of seizure that requires medical intervention? If you are unsure, ask your physician to help you set guidelines for the school staff.

They need to know the names of your child's medications. Your neurologist's office may be able to provide you with fact sheets about these medications to share with school personnel.

School personnel need to know the name and phone number of your neurologist. Many neurologists work with a nurse who can be a contact to the school nurse or health aide, answering questions about the seizures and medications. The school will ask you to sign a release of information so that they can contact your child's physician. If you do not want to sign a release for all school staff, have them identify one specified contact and one back-up contact that you will allow to call your physician's office.

They need to know when things change. If your child has developed a new seizure type, you need to provide the school staff with a description. If medications are being changed, you need to let the teacher know what effects this change may have on your child's ability to perform. The school needs to know if the effects will be temporary, improving as your child's body adjusts to the medication, or will be long term.

The Model Individual Education Plan (IEP) in Appendix A provides an overview for structuring your relationship with the school regarding your child's epilepsy.

▶ What if the school suggests restrictions for my child?
Some schools have a "policy" regarding epilepsy that fails to differentiate between the needs of children with various seizure types. Some schools have asked children to wear helmets during recess or limited the child's access to certain playground equipment. Some schools have refused to allow the child to participate in strenuous activities such as physical education class or exciting activities such as field trips, for fear of causing a seizure. Some schools have refused to allow the child to climb a flight of stairs for fear that if a seizure occurred, the child would be injured. While these restrictions sometimes may be appropriate, they are not appropriate for all children with epilepsy.

If your school has outlined restrictions for your child, discuss these restrictions with your neurologist. She can help you determine what restrictions, if any, are appropriate for your child. The neurologist can then provide a letter to the school administration indicating that inappropriate restrictions should be lifted.

▶ Does having epilepsy mean that my child will have problems with
   learning in school?
Children with epilepsy are at "increased risk" for learning problems. What does this mean? Risk refers to the chance that something will happen. Every child is at risk for learning problems, but for most children this risk is extremely low, meaning that it is unlikely that problems will occur. The odds

that a child with epilepsy will develop some type of learning problem are higher than for children without epilepsy. However, this does not mean that it will happen to *your* child.

We know from research that the risk of learning problems is related to a number of factors, including age of seizure onset, type of seizures, number of seizure types the child experiences, type and number of medications, and frequency of seizures. These factors are not independent. The type of medication chosen for your child is related to the type of seizures that your child experiences. The decision to treat seizures with more than one medication relates to your child's response to medication, to how disruptive the seizures are for your child, and to your child's risk for injury as a result of a seizure. Different types of seizures are likely to become evident at different ages. Your neurologist may be able to estimate your child's relative risk for learning problems.

Keep in mind that even if your child is at "high risk" for learning problems, he still will learn new things. The size of the steps taken in learning skills may be smaller. Your child may need more practice to learn and remember a skill. He may need certain kinds of material (more verbal description or more visual materials) in order to learn.

▶ **What kinds of learning problems might my child have?**
Learning problems come in many forms (See Table 4.1). Some children with epilepsy have subject-specific learning problems. Children with complex partial seizures are at increased risk for this type of learning problem. While the child does well in some subjects, one or two subjects are extremely difficult. If the child's overall ability to learn (intelligence IQ) falls within the average range, the subject-specific learning problems are referred to as a *learning disability*.

A learning disability reflects a relative weakness in some type of information processing. Information processing refers to how the child interprets what he sees or hears, not to how well the child sees or hears (acuity). If the weakness is in auditory processing, the child may have a disability that involves reading, spelling, or written language. If the weakness is in visual processing, the child may have a disability involving math or handwriting. Intervention involves teaching the problem subject in a different way than it is taught for most children (e.g., making reading more of a visual task, or math more of a verbal task).

If a child experiences a slower rate of learning in all subjects, this may reflect lower than average intelligence. Some schools refer to this as a *general*

TABLE 4.1

Comparison of Learning Disabilities and Mental Retardation

	Learning Disability	Mental Retardation
Intelligence	Average on either a measure of verbal or nonverbal reasoning skills (IQ score above 80)	Below average IQ on both verbal and nonverbal reasoning measures (IQ score less than 70)
Achievement	Average in some subjects	All academic skills are less well developed than other students of the same age; some skills may be better than others
Sensory impairment (inability to see or hear)	No	No
Exposure to education	Yes	Yes
Adaptive behavior (self-care and social skills)	Appropriate for age level	Delayed; child seems "immature"
Modifications need to support learning	Different approach to teaching for the problem subject (more visual or more verbal)	Slower rate of learning; more concrete explanation; direct teaching needed to generalize material

learning disability or *intellectual handicap.* When the learning problems are accompanied by delays in the development of self-care skills and social skills, the more appropriate term is mental retardation. *Mental retardation* refers to a slower rate of learning. It does not mean that a child is unable to learn. The child with mental retardation needs skills broken into smaller steps, with fewer steps presented at one time. He needs more repetition and practice to master the skills, and he may need direct teaching in how to use the skills in new situations, to generalize from one situation to another. Children with generalized tonic clonic seizures, with multiple seizure types, or with frequent, prolonged, poorly controlled seizures are at increased risk for mental retardation.

Children with epilepsy may have other special learning needs. Some children have difficulty with memory. Memory involves a number of steps, including initial encoding, transfer of the information to a long-term memory store, and finding the information again once stored. Seizures and medications can affect any or all steps in this process. Once the step(s) being affected have been identified, study strategies or methods for measuring learning can be modified to help the child. Some children with epilepsy experience brief lapses in consciousness that disrupt their attention. These children may need a study partner, closer supervision from the teacher, or to be allowed to tape record lectures. Many children with epilepsy process information more slowly than average. These children may need reduced assignments or extra time to complete assignments and tests in order to compete fairly with peers. Some children with epilepsy have difficulty with organization and planning, leading to problems with working independently. These children may need more structure from teachers and may require direct instruction in order to learn ways to stay organized.

▶ **How will I know if my child is having a problem?**
It is essential that you establish a good working relationship with your child's teacher. The teacher needs to know that you are interested in your child's work, and how this compares to other students. While visiting the classroom, look at the work posted in the room, so that you can get a sense of what other children are able to do. Be sure to look at all the children's work. It is normal to see a range of skills. You want to know if your child is within that range.

Talk with your child about school. You need to ask specific questions, such as "What did you do in reading today?" rather than general questions such as "What did you do in school today?" Does your child have enthusiasm for some subjects and not other ones? Does your child like to go to school?

Go over completed work that your child brings home. You can use the completed work to check on her understanding of the assignment.

Do homework with your child. You will learn a lot by having your child show you what she is supposed to be doing with assignments, or by having her explain directions to you.

Observe your child in activities with other children of the same age. Does your child pay attention as well as others? Does she relate well to peers? Does your child share the same interests as others? Does she seem as coordinated as her peers?

▶ **If the teacher says my child has a problem, what do I do?**

First, get more information from the teacher. Most often, teachers begin the conversation by providing you with their conclusion (e.g., "I think Johnny has a reading disability. "I think Susie has Attention Deficit/Hyperactivity Disorder."). Ask for a description. What has the teacher seen that has led her to draw this conclusion?

Find out when the teacher first noticed the problem. You want to know if the problem is getting better, worse, or staying the same. You need to know if the problem is evident throughout the school day. Ask what happens as a result of the problem. Does your child have other children doing written work for him? Is your child unable to read math story problems, but able to read his reading textbook? Does your child still have to do the math story problems even if he can not read?

Find out what the teacher has already tried. Has the teacher given your child some extra help, or referred her for remedial services? Did the teacher try any different ways of presenting the material that is hard for your child?

With this information in hand, you are now ready to talk to your child. Let her know that the teacher has concerns, and reassure her that you want to help make school go better for her. Ask your child what she thinks will make it better.

Your investigation may have provided you with the answer to how to help your child. If not, you may want to contact your neurologist with the information that you have collected. Provide the neurologist with an overview of the behavioral description, what has been tried, and your child's perceptions of the problem. The neurologist may recommend that you contact the school and request an evaluation of your child by the school's multidisciplinary team, or may refer her to a neuropsychologist for evaluation.

▶ **How will the school address my child's special learning or performance needs?**

Two federal laws may apply to getting your child's needs met in the school setting. The Individuals with Disabilities Education Act (IDEA) applies to all children who have special needs in order to achieve in school. Section 504 of the Rehabilitation Act of 1973 applies specifically to individuals with a physically handicapping condition. Educational needs related to your child's seizure disorder and/or medication effects may be met under either one of these laws. See Table 4.2 for a comparison of these two laws.

When your child is having learning problems, you, your child's neurologist, or his teacher can initiate the evaluation process under IDEA legislation. The first step in this process is for you to meet with school staff (multidisciplinary team) to discuss your child and what the school plans to do to better understand his special learning needs. An assessment plan will be generated describing what tests and classroom observations will be done. The school staff person responsible for each test or observation will be listed. This may include special education teachers, a school psychologist, a speech and language pathologist, an occupational therapist, and a physical therapist. A teacher may observe your child working in his classroom. The school social worker may meet with you to gather more information about your child. The school needs your permission to do this assessment.

When the assessment has been completed, you will meet with the multidisciplinary team to review the results. If your child is found to be eligible for services under IDEA, an Individual Educational Plan (IEP) will be written. This defines what services your child will receive, the goals that his teachers expect your child to accomplish with these services, and when his progress will be reviewed. The IDEA legislation states that you have the right to be involved in creating the IEP. This means that you can offer suggestions about the goals that you want to include and goals that you do not feel are appropriate for your child. The school needs your permission to provide the services identified in this plan.

IDEA is a federal law that has created an outline of the process through which children shall be identified as having special needs. Each state has passed legislation defining how this law will be carried out in that state. Your school system should be able to provide you with written information on the procedures in your state, as well as information about what you can do if you do not agree with the recommendations of the multidisciplinary team and/or IEP. Most states have parent advocacy groups that can help you learn about the laws in your state. If disagreements arise, these groups can help you locate a parent advocate—a parent who has been trained to help other parents resolve disputes with schools. The PACER Center in Minneapolis, Minnesota maintains a list of parent advocacy groups around the country. You can contact the PACER Center by phone at 952-838-9000 or through the Internet at *www.pacer.org*.

Section 504 of the Rehabilitation Act is used when your child requires some modification of the regular classroom, but does not require specialized

TABLE 4.2

A Comparison of the IDEA Act and Section 504
of the Rehabilitation Act of 1973. Adapted from Cohen [1]

	IDEA Act	Section 504
Purpose	Establishes guidelines for delivery of special education services	Establishes guidelines to prevent discrimination against individuals with disabilities in educational settings
Eligibility	Categories for service delivery are defined; state legislation further specifies test score patterns or other documentation needed to be eligible for each category	Eligibility defined in general terms related to the presence of a physical (medical) or mental condition that significantly affects performance of one or more major life activities
Funding	Schools eligible for federal and state funds to support service provision	Schools receive no additional funding to support modifications defined in the 504 plan
Testing	Requires staffing by a multidisciplinary team to define a testing plan; test results serve as the basis for determining eligibility for services	No formal testing is required as the basis for developing a 504 plan
Service provided	Special education, meaning a change in the rate of teaching or approach to teaching	No change in the rate of teaching or approach to teaching
Monitoring of service needs	Defines regular intervals for review of the Individual Educational Plan and for re-evaluation of the Special Education Placement	No time intervals are defined for reviewing the 504 plan

	IDEA Act	Section 504
Identifying children in need of services	Schools required to take an active role in identifying children who are in need of special education services	No obligation for school to identify children in need of educational modifications under this plan
Involvement of parents in development of intervention plan	Requires that parents be notified of meetings and be allowed to participate in the development of their child's testing plan and educational plan	Does not require parent participation in development of intervention plan
Least restrictive environment	Requires that the child's teaching occur, as much as possible, with other children who do not have disabilities	Requires that the child's teaching occur, as much as possible, with other children who do not have disabilities
System for resolving disagreements between parents and school	Defines a due process procedure; i.e., steps for resolving disagreements	Requires that a method is available of addressing and resolving disagreements, but does not define the actual procedure

1. Cohen M. SECTION 504 AND IDEA: Limited vs. Substantial Protections For Children with AD/HD and Other Disabilities. Chicago: Monahan and Cohen Law Firm, 1999.

services from teachers or therapists in addition to the classroom teacher. A 504 plan is written through a conference with your child's teachers and one or more other school representatives. It often addresses issues such as modifications in testing procedures (e.g., untimed tests, oral responding), classroom expectations (e.g., shortened assignments, reduced demands for copying from the blackboard), or access to adaptive equipment (e.g., computer use rather than handwriting).

▶ **How does a neuropsychologic assessment differ from the testing provided by the school?**

A neuropsychologist may use some of the same tests that are used by the multidisciplinary team in the school. School psychologists are interested in the resulting scores—that is, in how much skill your child demonstrates and how that compares to other children of the same age or grade. The neuropsychologist is interested in how your child achieved the scores. If your child does poorly on a task, neuropsychologic assessment is focused on breaking the task into components and attempting to identify what piece of the process is missing. When the neuropsychologist sees a weakness in a skill, she uses additional tests to try to identify why weaknesses are present.

The school psychologist is likely to have a standard battery of tests that are used for all children of your child's age who are referred to him. The neuropsychologist's experience with seizure disorders and the medications used to treat seizures provides him information that will help to predict where your child may have difficulty. She can then select tests sensitive to these problem areas.

The school psychologist looks at your child's pattern of performance on measures of intelligence and academic achievement, using this information to determine where your child may need help. She may talk to you about your child being an auditory or visual learner. The neuropsychologist looks at your child's pattern of performance in two ways. First, she uses information about the pattern of strengths and weaknesses to help define ways to use your child's strengths to help him compensate for areas of weakness. By having pursued the "why" for weaknesses, the neuropsychologist may be able to provide more detail for the team to use in identifying ways to help your child. Second, the neuropsychologist uses information about your child's seizure disorder and current pattern of performance to help identify areas that may become difficult in the future. Compensatory skills can be introduced before a problem develops rather than after your child has experienced failure.

▶ **If my child is having learning problems, should I go to a neuropsychologist instead of having my child seen by the school assessment team?**

The answer to this question depends on your child's individual needs. Your neurologist can help you make this decision. In addition, you may want to consider practical issues such as the speed with which your child will be seen by the school assessment team and whether or not your insurance will help to cover the cost of neuropsychologic assessment. The Model IEP in Appendix A summarizes testing approaches that the school staff can use to begin assessment of problem areas that occur frequently in children with epilepsy.

Your neurologist may recommend a neuropsychologic assessment in the following situations:

- Memory problems are suspected. While school psychologists have tasks that can screen memory skills, the neuropsychologist's tests provide more detail, determining if your child is having problems getting information into memory (storage) or is able to get the information filed in memory, but unable to find it (retrieval).
- It is suspected that medications and/or seizures are playing a role in your child's learning problems.
- A change in treatment for the seizures is planned. The neurologist may ask the neuropsychologist to use tests to establish a "baseline" so that the effect of the treatment on your child's continued development of specific skills can be measured. After the change in treatment, the neuropsychologist repeats the baseline tests to see if the treatment resulted in a change in skills.
- Your child has already been assessed by the school, but has not made progress in response to the teaching strategies identified and used as a result of that testing.
- Your child's seizures have a known cause. For most children with epilepsy, the reason for the seizures is not known. However, some children have seizures as a result of a *malformation* (a small part of brain that does not form correctly), as a result of a tumor, or as the result of damage to the brain such as a stroke or accident. The neuropsychologist's knowledge of the effects of these known causes on brain organization and skill development will allow him to better tailor his testing to your child's needs.

▶ **Does getting help for my child mean that she will be labeled for life?**
The IDEA legislation provides parents with the right to review their child's school file. The school has the right to have a staff person present during this review. If you find information in your child's file that is no longer accurate, you can ask to have this corrected. The school staff will either remove the information or mark it as no longer accurate.

For a child to be successful as an adult, she has to feel effective and that she can meet any challenges that occur. Untreated learning problems result in school failure, which in turn damages self esteem. While a child may be teased about getting special help, children are also teased about failing in school. If the child feels successful—has positive self esteem—she will be able to handle the teasing. Labeling your child in order to get the educational services that she needs is a small price to pay for supporting her self esteem.

▶ **Does Section 504 and IDEA apply if my child attends a private school?**

If your child attends a private or parochial school, he is still eligible for all of the services covered by IDEA. These services are available to him through the public school district in which you live. His classroom teacher, his neurologist, or you can contact the public school to have your child's educational needs reviewed by the multidisciplinary team. Your child is entitled to assessments by the therapists and psychologists employed by the public school. If he needs special education services, he can receive these services through the public school. However, the public school is not required to provide any of these services to him while he is in the private school's building. In other words, you may have to take your child to the public school for testing. The public and private school may need to work out a way for your child to get special education services at the beginning or end of the school day, moving between the public and private school setting.

Section 504 applies to any school that receives federal funding. A private school does not have to make the accommodations that a public school must make under Section 504. However, most teachers are committed to helping the children they teach. Most teachers are willing to make the accommodations that your child needs even if they are not required by law to do so.

If your child develops special educational needs while attending private school, it is important to weigh the advantages and disadvantages to continuing at the private school. Private schools often offer a smaller class size. What your child misses in special education service may be offset by what he gains in individual attention from the teacher. Friendships are another important consideration. If your child has met with acceptance and understanding in his current school setting, it may be best to keep him in that setting. It is helpful to make lists of the advantages and disadvantages offered in each setting when deciding if a change in schools is appropriate.

▶ **What about my dreams?**

All parents dream of their child growing up, getting a job, and establishing a life of his own. These dreams are challenged when mental retardation or severe learning disabilities occur. In some cases, dreams are shattered. Parents experience grief when dreams "die" just as people grieve over the death of a person. If your dreams are challenged, allow yourself time to grieve. It is a normal reaction. Recognize that grief may pop up repeatedly as your child grows to adulthood, often triggered by events that remind you of your old dreams. Build new dreams for your child. Every child achieves something.

The size of the steps, rate of progress, and final goal may be different from that of the average child, but the achievement is still worth celebration.

▶ **Taking epilepsy to school sounds like a difficult job.**
Helping children to do well in school is a big job for any parent. That job is more difficult when your child has a chronic health problem. When your child has a health problem that is often misunderstood, the job is even more challenging. But there is good news. You have the resources of the Epilepsy Foundation, your neurologist, and your neurologist's staff to aid you in educating the school. Federal and state laws guarantee your child's rights to a school program in the least restrictive environment that provides educational benefit. The "least restrictive environment" means that your child should be with his peers for all activities he is capable of doing with them. "Educational benefit" means that your child is making progress, and learning new things in response to the educational program. You will find teachers, speech pathologist, occupational therapists, physical therapists, psychologists, and neuropsychologists to work with you to help your child succeed during the school years.

Suggested Books for the Elementary Classroom

Dottie the Dalmatian Has Epilepsy. Gladstone, NJ: Tim Peters & Company, 1996.

Grosselin K. Taking Seizure Disorders to School. Valley Park, MO: JayJo Books, 1996.

Suggested Pamphlets Available from the Epilepsy Foundation

Teachers:

Epilepsy in Children: Learning and School Performance

The Teacher's Role: A Guide for School Personnel

Students:

Seizure Man: First Aid for Seizures. Bowman Grey Medical School.

Seizure Man: In the Classroom. Bowman Grey Medical School.

Spider-Man Battles the Myth Monster. Marvel Comics.

Effects of Focal Epilepsy:
A Guide to Brain Organization

CHAPTER 5

The Frontal Lobes

THE FRONT PART of the brain serves as a connection between our internal world and the world around us. The frontal lobes are connected to all other parts of the brain. They contain the motor pathways that allow us to respond to what is occurring around us. While other parts of the brain process and interpret sensory information, the frontal lobes determine what response is made to that information, organizes the response, executes it, and assesses the effect to determine if the response should be repeated in the future. While other parts of the brain are involved in storing information in memory, the frontal lobes are involved in retrieving that information and applying it to new situations. The frontal lobes play a role in determining where attention is focused and how long it stays focused. Frontal lobes control motor output, our means of demonstrating what we are thinking, feeling, and wanting to do.

The frontal lobes serve as a "secretary," keeping us organized and prioritizing what we need to do. They serve as a "project supervisor," organizing the approach for achieving a goal and making modifications in approach as we go along. The frontal lobes serve as a "parent" or "social monitor," making sure that behavior is appropriate in the current situation. These skills develop gradually during childhood and adolescence. When frontal lobes are not functioning properly, teachers may view the problems as "nothing more than immaturity," believing that the child will "grow out" of the problems.

▶ **What happens when the frontal lobes do not work properly?**
A variety of behaviors can occur when the frontal lobes do not function effectively. The specific set of problems you may see in your child are related to the specific areas of the frontal lobe that are not working well.

Controlling When to Respond

The frontal lobes help us decide when to respond. In some cases, dysfunction makes it hard for a child to start a response. He may be unable to find something to do, just sitting and doing nothing until prompted by his parent and helped to get involved in an activity. The child may know that he wants something, but make no effort to get it unless it is visible to him. Problems with initiation are less common than problems with stopping or inhibiting responses. When a child has problems stopping or inhibiting responses, this problem is called *disinhibition*.

Disinhibition can be evident through a child's language. Some children with frontal lobe dysfunction have difficulty keeping their thoughts to themselves. The child says whatever she is thinking. She may interrupt when others are speaking or change topic in the middle of a conversation. Comments may be triggered by sights, sounds, or events in the environment or may reflect the sudden overt expression of the child's ongoing train of thought. Frequently, comments are tangentially related to what is occurring. If you think about it, you can see how the child's thoughts related to something that she saw or heard. Other people may view resulting comments as socially inappropriate, such as a child commenting on someone's age or appearance.

Disinhibition can be evident through a child's actions. Some children with frontal lobe dysfunction are impulsive. The child acts before he has a chance to consider if the action is really a good thing to do. For example, the child may run into the street without looking just because he saw a friend on the other side. The child may go sharpen a pencil in the middle of the teacher's instructions. He may get up and run to the window because he hears a siren, even though he is in the middle of dinner. Impulsive children have difficulty delaying the meeting of a need, such as waiting to eat a meal if they happen to be hungry or waiting their turn to play a game.

Organizing How to Respond

The frontal lobes are responsible for generating problem solving strategies and organizing responses. While all young children engage in trial-and-error problem solving, children should become more systematic in their approach with age. Instead of repeating errors, the child becomes more aware of things she has already tried and avoids repeating errors. The next step in normal development involves learning to use language as part of the problem solving process. First, children will talk out loud, appearing to discuss options with themselves. Eventually, they learn to think about solutions, keeping the "talk" inside their heads. Children with frontal lobe problems may be stuck at the level of trial-and-error problem solving or may continue to talk out loud, rather than thinking about solutions. They do not appear to pay close attention to their work, fail to recognize an accurate action, and make the same mistake repeatedly. As a result, efforts to reach the desired goal are often met with frustration.

The frontal lobes are involved in sequencing a pattern of movements to achieve a specific goal. For example, the child with frontal lobe dysfunction may be told to "clean up your bedroom." While the child understands what a clean room looks like, he may have difficulty recognizing the steps he should take to achieve this goal. For example, he may stack toys on top of dirty clothes, only to then dump the stack of toys to pick up the dirty clothes. The frontal lobes are also involved in organizing language output, or sequencing thoughts in order to relate an event or information in an organized fashion. Children with problems that involve frontal lobe functions may relate bits of information, with the listener then faced with the problem of organizing and integrating it in order to understand what the child meant. In relating an event, the child may mix information from the ending with information from the beginning. Children with frontal lobe dysfunction may have trouble understanding the listener's perspective, assuming that the listener knows exactly what they are talking about. For example, a child may start telling a stranger about various family members without recognizing that the stranger does not know to whom the names refer.

Organization of visual scanning, such as moving from left to right to read, is a frontal lobe function. Most children learn to scan from left to right across a page, which is essential for reading. Children with frontal problems may skip words or lines in their scanning efforts. On worksheets, these children may jump around, completing whatever item catches their interest. They may turn in worksheets that are incomplete, failing to recognize that they missed some of the items.

Adapting Responses
Children with frontal lobe problems may fail to alter future responses based on the effect of a past response. They may repeat the same behaviors over and over again even though they are ineffective. For example, a child may repeatedly ask the same question even when she knows the answer. She may make a mistake in school work, erase the mistake, and make the same mistake again. This inappropriate repetition is called *perseveration*. In a sense, the child is "stuck in a rut" and needs help to develop a different behavior. Because of perseveration, children with frontal problems seem to show no

response to punishment for misbehavior, and are often described as failing to learn from their mistakes. Perseverative behavior can contribute to problems in accepting transitions (getting ready for school, changing to a different subject in school, stopping play to eat a meal). Such children may become upset when parents or teachers need them to shift from one behavior or activity to another. Often children with frontal problems are dependent on routine and become upset if the routine is interrupted or changes.

Regulating Emotions

Most of us are able to feel emotions with varying degrees of intensity. However, many children with frontal lobe problems experience emotions in an "all or none" fashion. They often demonstrate mood swings from very happy to very sad or very angry. The degree of emotional response seems out of proportion to the event that prompted it. Because of problems with perseveration and organization of responses, they may have difficulty finding a means for expressing their feelings that is both effective and socially acceptable.

Retrieving Information

The temporal lobes are involved in filing information in memory. The frontal lobes keep track of where information has been filed so that it can be retrieved. Children with frontal problems may sense that they know a piece of information, but be unable to think of it on demand. They may be able to recognize the information when presented with options, but be unable to recall it. Children with frontal dysfunction may have difficulty remembering the source of information. For example, if told to do two chores, the child may remember that he has two chores to do, but recall something that he was told to do yesterday rather than what he was told to do today.

Applying information

Children with frontal lobe problems are often effective at the rote learning of information—mastering isolated facts through repetition. However, they have difficulty in the flexible use of the information that they have learned. They may have trouble demonstrating skills if the materials used for demonstration are different from the materials used in learning. They may have difficulty in pulling information together from a variety of learning experiences and applying it to solve new problems. For example, a child may have difficulty using information to draw conclusions, to make comparisons and contrasts, or to make inferences. These skills become important in the junior high and senior high school years.

Paying Attention

Children with frontal lobe dysfunction may have difficulty deciding what is most important to pay attention to in the environment. Once focused, they may have difficulty keeping focused (poor concentration) or in shifting focus to something new.

▶ **Do the right and left frontal lobes have different functions?**

The brain is typically organized so that the left frontal lobe provides the organization for spoken language. This involves organizing words in appropriate sentence structure and sequencing thoughts in a logical order. The left frontal lobe controls the movements of the lips and tongue to produce speech sounds. It keeps track of where verbal material has been stored, helping to retrieve this information. It supports the flexible use of language. This includes being able to use context to assign the correct meaning to words that can mean more than one thing ("glasses" can refer to something that we drink from, or something we wear to improve vision). The left frontal lobe retrieves past learned verbal information, playing a role in combining the information as the basis for drawing new conclusions, making inferences, or making comparisons. These skills are referred to as higher order language functions.

The right frontal lobe serves similar functions for visual material. In addition, it plays an important role in directing attention and in regulating emotional expression. However, because the frontal lobes are so richly interconnected, seizures involving one frontal lobe tend to disrupt the functioning of both.

▶ **How do we help a child with frontal lobe problems?**

In general, your child's environment has to provide him with additional structure, that is, it has to serve as the secretary, project manager, and parent that your child cannot be for himself.

Providing Structure

It is important to have clear-cut general rules for specific situations. These rules need to be phrased in terms of what your child is expected to do. If you define what your child should not do, it is left up to him to think of an alternative. Your child may perseverate, producing the same incorrect behavior over and over again. Even if he thinks of a different response and uses it, the new action may be no better than the behavior you are trying to change. The rules defining what your child should do become the building blocks of structure. However, to be useful, these rules must be consistently enforced. Often it is helpful to post the household or classroom rules in a prominent location if your child can read or to frequently review them with the child if he cannot read. For children with limited reading skills, you can use drawings to prompt retrieval of the rules.

In the lower elementary grades, the teacher provides structure by telling the class exactly what to do, having the class immediately follow the direction, and then collecting the papers for grading. During the upper elementary years, teachers are preparing children for junior high. Assignments are often written on the blackboard. Worksheets are handed out. The child is given work periods, but is left to decide what work to complete. Completed work may not be collected until the next day. If work is not done, the child needs to remember to take all materials home, and to bring them back. Academic life often falls apart at this point for the child with frontal dysfunction.

Your child may need help in developing a structure that will allow him to cope with the organizational demands in the upper elementary and junior high levels. You and your child's teachers may need to teach him to use an assignment notebook. The notebook may need small squares in each assignment block for the child to use to check off work status (begun, completed, turned in) and a letter code for materials needed to complete the assignment. You may need to work with your child, experimenting with different types of notebooks and locker organizers to avoid "lost" work.

Developing Routines

Routines help your child to compensate for problems with organization. Initially, it may be necessary to use a notecard containing a verbal or picture outline of the steps involved in a routine, allowing the child to check off each step as it is completed. As he masters the routine, steps will flow in sequence, with recall of each step prompted by acting on the preceding one. Routines are helpful for recurrent activities such as getting ready for school, entering or leaving school, doing homework, or going to bed. Routines can help the child prepare for and make the transitions that occur in his day.

TABLE 5.1

DESIGNING A BEHAVIOR SHAPING PROGRAM

1. Make a list of all behaviors that are a concern to you. Prioritize the list, selecting no more than two behaviors to work on at any given time.

2. For each target behavior, write a behavioral definition of what the child is doing now, and a definition of the goal behavior you want the child to demonstrate.

3. Define small intermediate steps, each step more closely approximated the desired goal.

4. As the child demonstrates the target behavior, interrupt her and prompt the next more appropriate behavior.

5. As the child learns the new behavior remind her of it as she enters situations in which the target behavior occurred.

6. When the new behavior is consistently evident, move to the next step in the shaping paradigm.

Organizing output

Structure, routines, and behavioral shaping (see Table 5.1) will help your child to develop patterns that organize behavioral output. To help him organize language output, you can provide him with questions that will elicit the information in a sequenced manner. As children reach the upper elementary grades, they are expected to generate organized written work, such as a book report or research paper. It may be helpful to teach your child to brainstorm, listing each possible idea for inclusion in the report on a separate notecard. He can then sort the notecards into stacks by topic, sequence the topics within each stack, and then sequence the topic stacks to proceed in a logical order. You can review the ideas with your child, asking him questions about main ideas and helping him add detail (recorded on the appropriate notecard). This notecard stack becomes your child's outline for the written report.

If your child has problems organizing language, he may benefit from doing written work on a computer. As with brainstorming, this allows the child to generate ideas freely. He can then review his writing, using word processing features such as cut/paste to organize the material.

In addition to having problems organizing written language, children with frontal lobe problems may have difficulty organizing a strategy to use in performing tasks based on the teacher's directions. Typically, teachers check a child's comprehension of directions by having him repeat them. The child with frontal dysfunction may be able to repeat directions, but still have little idea of how to organize actions to carry them out. If your child is slow to begin work, it is helpful to have him demonstrate what he thinks he should be doing as a check on his comprehension of directions.

Responding to Perseveration
When perseveration occurs in behavior such as persisting in an incorrect problem solving strategy, it is often necessary to stop your child, then direct her into a more appropriate response. When verbal perseverative behavior occurs, this can be dealt with either by teaching a routine (posting the answer to a perseverative question in a specific spot and directing your child to it) or by introducing a new topic.

Easing Transitions
Implementing a structured routine for the day helps to reduce problems in making transitions. For some children, it is helpful to make a written schedule or picture schedule of the day. The child can check the schedule throughout the day, preparing for upcoming changes. For young children, the picture schedule depicts the sequence of important events. For older children, words can be paired with time intervals, much like an adult's day planner. Some parents and schools have made laminated pieces for the schedule, using Velcro™ to attach pieces to the schedule board. This has two advantages. First, the child can remove each piece as the event is completed as part of a transition routine to the next event. Second, it allows for changes in schedule that may occur (occupational therapy occurring only on Tuesday, art on Wednesday and Friday).

Whether or not your child is using a schedule, it is also useful to warn him of a transition before it occurs. To help the child learn to use warnings to prepare for change, it is helpful to provide more than one warning ("In five minutes, it will be time to . . . ", "Finish up because in two minutes you will need to . . . ").

Reducing Emotional Lability
The key to reducing negative emotional outbursts is *prevention*. The amount of frustration in your child's day can be reduced by providing clear structure, routines, help in generating strategies when the initial approach fails, and warnings regarding transitions. As frustration declines, the amount of negative emotion experienced by your child also decreases. You may be able to rec-

ognize signs of building frustration, and help the child take a break from the activity (time away) or to move to a different activity before a negative outburst occurs. You may be able to suggest and prompt the use of appropriate means for feeling expression, helping her vent the feeling before an outburst occurs. Once loss of control is evident, it is best to allow time for your child to regain emotional control (time out), then redirect her back to whatever expectations were present at the time of the outburst.

Building Appropriate Behaviors
Negative consequences for misbehavior are ineffective for children with frontal lobe problems. Negative consequences tell your child what *not* to do, but do not help him to identify and shift to a better behavior. In addition, misbehavior may occur impulsively, without your child considering consequences at the time he acts. It is more effective to change behavior by building appropriate behaviors. For children with frontal dysfunction, it is necessary to work on the gradual building, prompting, and rewarding of the behavior that you want to see. For some behaviors, this takes *shaping*, a procedure in which you define your long term goal, then set up a series of steps that gradually move you from current behavior to this goal (see Tables 5.1 and 5.2). Each step is then prompted and practiced until mastered.

For some behaviors, the use of role playing to practice the behavior and prompting of the behavior's use is effective. For role playing, you recreate the problem situation and practice the desired behavior with your child through pretend play. As the child enters the real-life situation, you would remind him of the behavior that you have practiced together.

Supporting Information Retrieval
The memory system is like a filing system. If information is always rehearsed in the same way and with the same materials, it is stored in a single file related to that way of learning and that set of materials. If information is learned using more than one sense, practiced with a variety of materials, and related to previously learned information, then multiple files are established and cross-referenced. For children who have problems retrieving information from memory, it is important to teach information in a multisensory fashion, using both visual and verbal material. It is important to practice skills in more than one way, and with a variety of materials. This increases the number of ways through which your child can find the information. For example, spelling words can be practiced by dictating words to the child or by giving her all the letters for the word and having her sequence the letters.

TABLE 5.2

A Behavior Shaping Program to Reduce Aggressive Outbursts

Step 1: As the child becomes aggressive, interrupt him, physically placing the child in his bedroom for time out.

Step 2: As the child becomes aggressive, verbally prompt him to go to his bedroom.

Step 3: As the child begins to lose his temper, prompt him to take "time away" by going to his bedroom.

Step 4: As the child begins to lose his temper, prompt him to take "time away by going to his bedroom. As the child calms down, join him in the bedroom and practice counting to 10, while taking a few deep breaths to release tension.

Step 5: As the child begins to lose his temper, prompt him to take "time away" in his bedroom, counting to 10 and taking deep breaths to calm down once there.

Step 6: When the child can regain emotional control in the bedroom using counting and breathing, prompt him to use these skills as soon as he begins to lose his temper (dropping out "time away").

Step 7: As the child becomes engaged in a conversation or situation that typically results in loss of emotional control, prompt him to use counting and breathing to maintain control.

Step 8: The child can recognize the need to use counting and breathing to maintain control.

You could play "Hangman" with your child using the spelling words or create a multiple choice test in which the correct spelling is paired with another real word and a misspelled option. Some of these approaches place greater demands on language skills (sounding the word out as it is spelled) while others focus on recognizing the visual configuration of the word.

If your child has retrieval problems, she needs to learn to use *active learning strategies*. Active learning strategies also help to compensate for deficits in attention and concentration. *The goal of active learning strategies is to get your child to use the information as she is learning it.* The comprehension of reading material, can be improved by teaching your child to identify topic sentences, using the topic sentence to predict the paragraph's content, then reading to check the accuracy of the prediction. Taking notes as one reads provides a comprehension check as well as converting the language meaning into visual information.

The means for testing knowledge also vary in terms of the demands made on information retrieval. Many children with frontal problems that involve retrieval problems demonstrate learning best on multiple choice, true/false, and matching tests, rather than on tests that require information reproduction (fill-in-the-blank, short answer, essay). Modifications in the approach to testing can be made as part of a 504 plan.

Supporting Generalization of Learning

As children grow older they are asked to apply previous learning to new situations. Reading comprehension questions and test questions in applied subjects require the child to make comparisons, make inferences, and draw conclusions. Children with frontal dysfunction may have difficulty performing this mental operation. However, you can help your child to "bridge the gap" between facts learned and these higher order language operations. To "bridge the gap," ask the child a series of more concrete factual questions to help him gather the information that he needs to answer the more abstract question. For example, imagine that a social studies class has studied climate and economy in Alaska and in Alabama. A study guide question might ask: "Why don't they grow cotton in Alaska?" You or your child's teacher can help him by having him list information about climate and soil conditions in each state, then list the conditions needed to grow cotton. Once the lists are made, your child can compare the lists to arrive at the answer. Through repeated practice in this procedure, your child will learn a strategy for attacking such questions on his own.

Focusing Attention

If your child has problems focusing attention, you need to create an environment that supports attention to relevant information and reduces distractions. In the school setting, this can be accomplished through preferential seating at the front of the classroom and near a wall, reducing the number of distractions between your child and the teacher. Keeping your child's workspace clear of materials not needed for the task at hand is also important. A line guide that blocks the rest of the page can be used to keep focus on a single line of work at one time, while supporting tracking across the page. Using highlighters to draw attention to key information (changes in directions, signs for operations in math, subtle differences between similar words in reading and spelling) may be useful. In the upper grades, students can be given highlighted textbooks to help them focus learning efforts on the most relevant information.

Disinhibition

When children are verbally disinhibited, their comments can significantly disrupt classroom instruction. If your child frequently interrupts, you and the teacher can develop a gestured cue for your child to indicate that she needs to stop and wait. Often teachers will simple raise a hand, palm facing the child to signal "stop." Your child will learn to stay quiet while the hand is raised. When the teacher has completed what she is saying, she lowers the hand, allowing your child to make her comment. Structure and routines help your child when disinhibition involves actions rather than words.

▶ **Since the frontal lobes are important for social functioning, how can I help my child to have friends?**

Children with frontal dysfunction do best in structured social situations, those that are typically supervised by an adult and organized to achieve a goal. For example, participating in team sports is a structured social situation. Organizations such as scouting, 4-H, or church youth groups are structured social situations. "Hanging out" at a friend's house is an unstructured situation, while playing a video game with a friend is a structured social situation.

Children with frontal dysfunction can be helped to develop appropriate social routines through participation in a social skills or friendship group. In some schools, these groups are run by the school counselor or school social worker. In such a group, your child is taught what to say and what to do in a number of common social situations. She is given supervised practice using the skills within the group. While other children may be able to automatically apply these skills to everyday situations, your child may need prompting to use the behavior until the new skills become habit.

▶ **What is the single most important general principle in behavioral intervention when frontal lobe problems are present?**

Interventions work by helping your child to compensate for skills that are not developed to an age-appropriate level. Interventions do not cause the skill deficit to disappear. Often, people are tempted to discontinue an intervention as soon as a child improves, only to learn that he needs the intervention in place to support that improvement. You are teaching your child routines.

Interventions supporting these routines need to be gradually tapered rather than abruptly stopped.

▶ What about medication?

Children with frontal lobe dysfunction may benefit from medications targeted to some of their symptoms. Medications can help to support the focusing and sustaining of attention, and to reduce frequent mood swings. Medications can also help to reduce perseverative behavior, helping the child to tolerate the transitions that are part of everyday living. Medications may affect how fast the body breaks down and uses an antiepileptic drug (AED). If you feel that behavior-based or environment-based interventions are not working for your child, discuss the use of psychoactive medications with your neurologist. She may refer you to a child psychiatrist to manage this aspect of treatment.

▶ What about my feelings?

Children with frontal lobe deficits can be confusing, frustrating, or embarrassing for a parent. It is important to distinguish those things over which you have control from those things over which you have no control.

As a parent, you have some control over the amount of structure and routine in your child's day and over the situations the child encounters in a day. How your child reacts to the experiences she encounters within the day is beyond your control. Whether or not misbehavior occurs is beyond your control. You *do* have control over how you react to misbehavior and the attempts you make to teach appropriate behaviors. Your child's reactions to your interventions are beyond your control. If you set small goals for you and your child, you both will experience success. If you expect to eliminate your child's special needs, both of you will experience frustration and defeat.

▶ Who will help me with my child?

Children with frontal dysfunction may show some, but seldom all, of the potential problems discussed in this chapter. If your child has seizures arising from the frontal lobes, neuropsychologic assessment can help you to understand what specific problems he is experiencing. The neuropsychologist can help you to identify strategies to help your child as he progresses through school. Depending on your child's age at the time of testing, the neuropsychologist can help you identify areas of risk for future problems so that you and the school staff can watch for and plan for these potential problems.

Clinical psychologists differ in their approaches to treatment. If your child is having behavior problems in the context of frontal dysfunction, a psychologist specializing in behavioral therapy can help you to develop shaping programs for him. Traditional talk-type psychotherapy, in which insight into behavior is expected to produce behavior change is ineffective for children with frontal dysfunction. Your neurologist or a child psychiatrist can help to select appropriate medications to address problems with emotional control and attention.

CHAPTER 6

The Temporal Lobes

▶ **What do the temporal lobes do?**

For most people, each temporal lobe has a special job to do. Both temporal lobes process sounds, interpreting what we hear. For most people, the left temporal lobe specializes in understanding and contributing to the production of language. The right temporal lobe is involved in processing sound patterns that become music, or the changes in vocal quality that help to express feelings and intentions. For people who are left-handed or who have experienced damage to the left temporal lobe early in life, language may be controlled by the right side of the brain or by both sides. For the purpose of this chapter, we talk about skills based on typical brain organization; that is, left hemisphere control of language.

The left temporal lobe interprets the sound patterns that make up words, associating these patterns with meaning (*listening comprehension*). The left temporal lobe works together with the *parietal lobe* to associate the visual pattern of words with meaning, or the sequence of letter sounds with meaning, allowing us to understand what we read. The left temporal lobe works together with the frontal lobes to produce language. While the frontal lobe controls the motor movements involved in speech, connections between temporal and frontal structures are important in the organization of what is said (*oral expression*). In essence, this interconnected system organizes a series of thoughts into a logical sequence and puts each thought into a correct form so that others understand (sentence structure and grammar).

The right temporal lobe interprets musical patterns. It also interprets the changes in word emphasis and tone of voice that communicates the speaker's intentions or emotions (*prosody*). For example, the words "that is pretty" can be a question or a statement. The speaker's pattern of emphasis on words makes the difference.

The right temporal lobe works with the right frontal lobe when we attempt to reproduce what we see. It is responsible for spatial organization when we draw or use other materials to construct an image of what we see. To understand spatial organization, let's think about drawing a tree. First, you would analyze the tree. You identify the parts, such as the roots, trunk, branches, and leaves. As you draw the tree, the temporal lobe plays a role in locating parts with respect to one another (the roots come out of the bottom of the trunk, the branches come out of the top). The temporal lobe tells you "where in space" each part goes. Together with the frontal lobe, a pattern of movements is generated to implement the spatial plan.

The temporal lobe curls inward, somewhat like the appearance of a snail shell. The curled portion that rests near the middle of the brain plays a very important role in memory. It is called the mesial temporal lobe. This area includes structures called the *amygdala* and the *hippocampus*. The amygdala is involved in making the automatic associations between things we experience in our world that produce pain or emotional reactions and the resulting reactions that occur. For each of us, certain things produce feelings of fear (snakes, thunderstorms), feelings of happiness (seeing family members), and feelings of contentment (the smell of fresh baked cookies). The amygdala is involved in learning these associations from a series of experiences (helping us remember that touching the hot stove produces pain). We don't have to think about these associations—the feeling comes to mind whenever we encounter the sight, sound, or smell that is part of the association. Case reports of individuals sustaining damage to the right amygdala suggests that this structure is important in our ability to remember faces—to recognize that we have seen someone before.

We also have a memory system that is involved in learning "facts" such as school information, people's names, the way to get to the grocery store, and the phone message that you are supposed to deliver. We can think of this memory system as if it were a large filing cabinet. The *mesial* temporal lobes do two jobs in the memory process. First, they temporarily hold information in mind, allowing us to repeat back what we have just heard or to copy what we just saw. The hippocampus is essential for the next step in the memory system—moving this temporary information into a more permanent memory store. In essence, the hippocampus helps to file the information. The frontal lobes of the brain keep track of where the information has been filed and play a role in retrieving the information when we need it later. The left hippocampus specializes in filing verbal information while the right hippocampus specializes in filing visual and spatial information. If one hippocampus is injured, the remaining hippocampus takes over its functions.

▶ **What happens when the left temporal lobe is not working properly?**
When seizures or injury affects the left temporal lobe, a child may have problems with understanding what is said to him (receptive language). The child may recognize that a word is familiar, but be unable to remember what it means. He may have problems related to the rate of speech. In other words, he can understand when someone speaks slowly, but can't keep up when the person speaks quickly. The child may have problems with sentence structure. He may be able to understand short simple sentences, but get lost in sentences that are long and contain clauses. Passive sentence structure is particularly challenging to children with temporal dysfunction ("The boy pushed the girl in the wagon.") The child may have difficulty learning and understanding language concepts, abstract words that describe the qualities of objects (big/little; same/different), location of objects (behind, next to), relative quantity (more/less), and sequence of actions (before/after, first/last). Problems with language comprehension may be misinterpreted as other types of problems. Teachers or parents may think that the child is not paying attention or is easily distracted because he does not follow directions. Parents or teachers may think that the child is being oppositional or disobedient, seeing him as having a behavior problem rather than realizing that he has a language problem. The same type of problems with language comprehension can occur for reading as well as for understanding spoken language.

When the left temporal lobe is not working properly, children often demonstrate problems with word retrieval (also called *word finding* difficulty). Everyone has had the experience of starting to talk about someone and suddenly being unable to remember that person's name, that is a word finding problem. This occurs more frequently in children with temporal lobe damage. The child may begin a sentence, then suddenly "get stuck," being unable to recall the next word. The words that give children trouble are usually names for something (people, objects, concepts). Sometimes the child produces a word that is similar to the word for which he is looking. Sometimes the child produces a word that sounds similar to the one that he wants, but it is not really a word at all. Often children will use a gesture, description, or a vague term ("thing") to substitute for the word that they can't recall. Some children simply give up, telling others to "never mind," in response to the frustration of word finding problems. When children are experiencing significant problems with word finding, they may choose not to speak rather than to work through the frustration of speaking. Parents or teachers may interpret this behavior as signs of shyness or social withdrawal.

When the left mesial temporal lobe is not working properly, the child may have difficulty remembering verbal information long enough to use it. For example, if given a direction, the child may be able to repeat it, but he loses track of the information as he attempts to turn it into a sequence of actions for following the direction. Children may also have difficulty moving information into longer term memory storage. Children with mesial temporal lobe problems often need to work harder than other children to learn new information. They may need to practice the information more often when learning it. Children with mesial temporal dysfunction may seem to understand a new concept as it is taught one day, but forget it by the next day. Once the concept is learned, the child may need to review information frequently so that it is not forgotten.

▶ **What happens when the right temporal lobe is not working properly?**
Children with right temporal dysfunction may have problems interpreting the vocal pattern that is essential for understanding prosody. They may fail to realize that parents are becoming angry with them until the parent shows anger through physical signs or puts the angry feeling into words. They may fail to realize that people are joking with them, taking their comments seriously. When the right temporal lobe is not working properly, the child may have difficulty copying drawings or visual patterns. She can see the details accurately, but has trouble organizing and sequencing movements to reproduce what is seen. If shown a complex design, the child may draw all of the parts, but fail to align them as they were presented in the design. Children with right temporal dysfunction may have difficulty producing "neat" handwriting, failing to space appropriately between letters within words and between words when printing. They may also produce writing that is inaccurately placed with respect to the lines on the paper.

Right mesial temporal structures are believed to be involved in memory for visual information such as faces, designs, and locations. Children with dysfunction involving the right mesial temporal lobes may have difficulty learning the basic association between letter symbols and letter names. The child may have difficulty recalling locations on a map, or remembering steps in a skill that was demonstrated but not described. For example, the child may be attentive to the teacher as she demonstrates a multistep math procedure, but find that she is unable to reproduce the same sequence when trying to complete her worksheet. Deficits in visual memory are more difficult to measure because most materials for visual memory tests can be described with words. If a child performs adequately, the examiner cannot tell from the child's performance if this was because the child remembered what she saw, or was very effective in describing the information to herself and remembering that description.

▶ **What can you do to help your child?**

Language Comprehension
A speech and language pathologist has special training to help individuals who have language comprehension problems. The speech and language pathologist can provide therapy to help improve your child's language comprehension. They can also give you suggestions that will help your child to cope with the comprehension problems.

Language comprehension problems are most often noticed because a child has difficulty with following directions. Parents are left wondering if their child did not understand them, or just did not want to do what she was asked to do. There are some simple practical things that you can do to support your child's understanding you. First, get the child's full attention. Turn off the television or other sources of competing sound. Make sure that she has stopped what she was doing and is looking at you. Second, watch your rate of speech. It is important to talk slowly, allowing pauses after key words so that she has a chance to assign meaning to what you have just said before you go on to say more. Third, keep it short. If you are telling your child to do more than one thing, you can support her understanding by giving the direction and then repeating just the key words ("Go upstairs, brush your teeth, then put on your pajamas. Upstairs, teeth, then pajamas."). Gestures that demonstrate your meaning will also be helpful.

For some children, problems with remembering what is said (a *verbal memory deficit*) affect comprehension. For these children, you can construct picture or word checklists (depending on reading level) to outline the steps for everyday directions. Checklists for recurring routines (daily chores, bedtime and morning routine) can be laminated so that they can be used, wiped clean, and used again. For tasks that only happen once in a while, a wipe-off slate can be used for the checklist. It is important to involve your child involved in creating the checklist. This will teach her a *compensatory mechanism* for her language comprehension and memory problems. Compensatory mechanisms are skills your child uses to "get around" the problem.

How do you know if your child has understood you? Most parents ask a child to repeat back what she was told to do. However, your child may be able to repeat your words without really understanding how to turn those words into actions that will allow her to complete the task. If you suspect that your child has comprehension problems, or you want to make sure you were understood, ask your child to show you what she was asked to do. If she can't do this, you know that you need to provide more explanation before she will be able to complete the task on her own.

In the early school years, most teaching is done in a multisensory fashion. In other words, the teacher uses words, demonstration, and pictures to communicate with children. Some children with language comprehension problems do well in the early school years because of the presence of these visual cues. However, teaching becomes more language-based in the upper elementary years, as teachers begin to teach primarily through lectures and class discussion. In the secondary grades, children are expected to take notes on lecture material. Children with left temporal dysfunction may not be able to comprehend the material at the teacher's rate of speech. It is helpful to provide these children with a tape recorder so that they can listen to sections of lecture where they became lost. Children with comprehension problems may not be able to listen to the teacher and take notes at the same time, finding that each of these tasks requires their full attention. Children with right temporal dysfunction may not be able to write fast enough or the resulting notes may be illegible. The school can be asked to provide an assigned note taker (another student whose notes are photocopied for your child) or to provide your child with a copy of the teacher's notes. These modifications can be made as part of a 504 plan.

Word Finding

Word finding problems are frustrating. Think about what is like to know what you want to say, but to be unable to say it. When your child is "stuck" on a word, it is very tempting to just say the word for him. However, some of the time you will not be sure of what your child was intending to tell you. Some children will be embarrassed or angry when this type of help is given. A speech and language pathologist can help him find a strategy to compensate for word finding problems. For some children, it is best to encourage them to use description, "talking around the word." Often this process helps them remember the word. Even if it doesn't help your child recall the word, he will still be able to get his meaning across. Gestures can also be helpful in getting the meaning across, reducing the child's frustration at not being understood. Some children find that it is most helpful to run through the alphabet in their mind. The beginning sound of the word may be enough to help the child recall the word.

If your child has frequent word finding problems, you want to stay alert to the kinds of tests being used in school to assess learning. Fill-in-the-blank tests or questions requiring single words or short phrases for answers underestimate your child's actual learning. You can ask the school to provide your child with a word list for these types of tests (word bank), turning the test into a matching task. Use of true/false or multiple-choice tests also provides a fair estimate of learning. In some cases, schools have allowed a child to use his notes or to take the test in an open book fashion. These accommodations are frequently made in schools as part of a 504 plan, but you may need to ask for them.

Memory Problems

When memory problems are the result of mesial temporal dysfunction, your child will have difficulty *encoding* information; that is, getting information moved into more permanent memory stores. Problems can involve *memory capacity*—the amount of information stored at one time, and/or *encoding speed*—the number of repetitions needed to get the information into memory stores.

There are two general approaches to helping children with capacity problems. First, the amount to be remembered can be reduced by embedding it in a meaningful context. It is much harder to remember a list of words (dog…brown…the . . .sleepy . . .is) than to remember a sentence (The brown dog is sleepy). The meaning unites the words so that they can be stored as two bits of information (brown dog, sleepy) rather than as five bits of information. For school work, we can provide a meaningful context by relating material to pictures in the textbook, by reducing description to an outline or flow chart, or by talking about new information in the context of previous learning or experiences. Creating a mnemonic reduces information. For example, the mnemonic for remembering the lines in music in treble clef is "**E**very **G**ood **B**oy **D**oes **F**ine" and the mnemonic for treble clef spaces is "F..A..C..E." When capacity is a problem, long lists of items can be learned more effectively by being broken into shorter lists. For example, if a child needs to learn ten spelling words per week, she can focus on five of the words the first night, then the other five the next night, combining the lists as words are mastered.

When the child has problems with speed of encoding, the best answer is to provide more rehearsal. It is most effective to space the practice out over the course of the day. For example, a middle school student needing to learn vocabulary words for a science class can make flashcards of the words and definitions, then practice the flashcards during breaks throughout the school day. Rather than spending an hour studying spelling words the night before the test, the child may do better with 20 minutes of practice every night for three nights.

Memory skills are important in life at home as well as at school. Interventions for the home are related to a child's age. For preschool age children, parents need to provide frequent reminders of things to remember. The parent may find it less frustrating to give the child single-step directions, having him come back as each is completed rather than attempting to get him to remember a two-step direction. For elementary school age children, the use of checklists is recommended. Once a child can read and write, parents should start expecting the child to keep a notebook with him or to write things on a calendar, then check the calendar each day. A pill box arranged by day and dose, coupled with a watch with an alarm can help older children with memory problems become independent in taking medication.

Memory problems may be restricted to certain kinds of material. Children may be good at encoding what they hear, but poor at remembering what they see, or vise versa. When encoding problems are modality-specific, the child can compensate by converting material to the strong modality. Verbal material can be converted to visual material by making flow charts, making time lines for history events, and associating content with pictures in the textbook. When memory for visual material is affected, the child can be encouraged to use words to describe the material. For example, in learning the location of countries on a map, the child can talk about countries being "above," "below," "to the right of," and "to the left of " a single country. Math operations are often taught through demonstration. Children with visual memory problems can be helped to generate an outline for the operation, using a phrase to describe each move with the spatial array of the math problem.

Prosody

Children who have difficulty understanding prosody need to directly ask others when they are unsure of the other's intentions. The parents, siblings, and friends of children with problems interpreting prosody need to use words, not tone of voice, to get their meaning across ("I am getting angry with you." "I mean it. Do it now.") Children with deficits in comprehension of prosody can be taught to use "body language," such as changes in facial expression, to help them interpret meaning. Situation cues can also be helpful.

Drawing/Construction

During the early elementary grades, children often demonstrate learning through coloring and construction tasks. Children with right temporal dysfunction can become frustrated when their work does not match their knowledge. For children who have poor control in coloring and handwriting, teachers can be asked to grade work in subjects other than handwriting based on the child's content rather than considering "neatness" as part of the child's grade. Children who print or write slowly can have assignments shortened or be given extra time to complete them. As children progress into the mid-elementary years, they are often expected to copy information from the blackboard or from textbooks. Children who print or write slowly can have this information given to them rather having to copy it. These modifications can be made in school as part of a 504 plan for your child.

Printing places greater demands on spatial organization than does writing in cursive. In cursive, the child needs to make a spatial decision between words. In printing, the child has to make a spatial decision for the placement of each letter. As a result, there may be as much space or more space between letters within words as there is between words. The child can be taught to place his little finger at the end of a word, starting the next word on the right side of the finger. As he progresses into the upper elementary years, he can be taught computer keyboarding to compensate for handwriting problems.

▶ **Who will help my child?**

When children's seizures involve the temporal lobes, a neuropsychologic assessment is a good starting point to identify your child's relative strengths and weaknesses. The goal of this assessment is twofold. First, it will help you to understand your child's skills. You will get an idea of what is fair to expect from her. You may find that what you suspected were problems with inattention or with bad behavior actually have another source. Having accurate information will allow you to be more supportive of your child and less frustrated with her. Second, the pediatric neuropsychologist will help you determine what you should do for areas of relative weakness. If weaknesses involve receptive or expressive language, the neuropsychologist will recommend that you arrange treatment for your child from a speech and language pathologist. If she has weaknesses that involve spatial organization, the neuropsychologist may suggest that your child work with an occupational therapist. If memory problems are present, the neuropsychologist will help you to identify strategies that you and your child can use to help her compensate for these problems.

The neuropsychologist can give you the information that you need to work with your child's school to meet her educational needs.

Children with language-based learning problems are at increased risk for problems with anxiety and depression. By identifying problems early and providing your child with appropriate treatment, you may be able to reduce this risk. If your child shows the warning signs of anxiety or depression (see Tables 10.2 and 10.3) a pediatric psychologist or clinical psychologist can help.

CHAPTER 7

The Occipital and Parietal Lobes

▶ **What do the occipital lobes do?**

The *occipital lobes* are located at the back of the brain. The eyes send information to the occipital lobes. The occipital lobes register the characteristics of what we see and then send the information on to the *parietal lobes* for interpretation. For example, the occipital lobe determines that we are looking at a colored round object. The parietal lobe determines that it is a red ball, not an orange or a globe. The left occipital lobe receives information about the right half of what we see (right visual field); the right occipital lobe receives information about the left half of what we see (left visual field).

▶ **What happens when seizures arise from the occipital lobes?**

When you slip and fall on the ice, hitting the back of your head, you may see moving bright dots of light (seeing "stars"). This is because you have jarred the occipital lobes. When focal seizures occur in an occipital lobe, the child may report similar sensations, seeing colors, lights, or a pattern. Because each occipital lobe receives information from only one visual field, the child may report that the things she sees are off to the right or to the left. If occipital lobe seizures result from actual damage to one side of the brain, the child may also have a visual field defect, and be unable to see information to the right side or the left side. The child can be taught to compensate by turning her head. In a sense, she moves the information into the intact visual field.

Because the occipital lobe is the first stopping off point for visual information, when the occipital lobe is not working properly, the parietal lobe may not receive the information it needs to function properly. The problems that may result and the things you can do to help your child with these problems are discussed below.

▶ What do the parietal lobes do?

The main job of the parietal lobes is to put sensory information together. Sounds are initially received in the temporal lobe. Visual information is initially received in the occipital lobe. Information from touch (pain, temperature, texture, movement) is initially received in an area in the parietal lobe where it meets the frontal lobe. In these *primary sensory reception areas*, the brain recognizes that sensation has occurred. The parietal lobe puts all of the sensory information together and assigns meaning to it. While the occipital lobe receives information about facial features, the parietal lobe determines if it is a familiar or unfamiliar face and whether the face is happy, sad, angry, or showing no emotion at all. While the temporal lobe receives information about sound, the parietal lobe puts the information together with our knowledge of words to assign meaning to the sound pattern. The parietal lobe may determine that the sound pattern is a word, a song, or an environmental sound such as a door bell or a passing car. When a child looks at a word, tracing the letters of a word with his finger as he sounds it out, the parietal lobe puts this information together to identify the word and its meaning (reading).

▶ What happens when the parietal lobes are not working properly?

When the right parietal lobe is not working properly, the child will have problems interpreting what he sees. He may have difficulty breaking visual information into components (*spatial analysis*) or putting visual information together into a single meaningful whole (*visual integration*). These skills are important in two areas of life. First, visual processing skills contribute to handwriting and to artistic ability. When the right parietal lobe is not working properly, the child may have difficulty learning to write neatly. He can form letters, but the letters may vary in size and may drift above or below the line. The child may do poorly at solving puzzles. He may have little interest in building with blocks because the structures do not come out looking right. Drawing, coloring, and cutting skills may be less well developed than for other children of the same age.

Second, visual processing skills contribute to social functioning. The words "I love you" can have many different meanings depending on body language, facial expression, tone of voice, and the situation in which they are spoken. We use spatial analysis skills to interpret various facial expressions (questioning look versus a happy excited look) and body positions (leaning in close versus shrugging shoulders and walking away). We use visual integration skills to put these observations together in the context of the situation. When seizures disrupt the right parietal lobe, the child may have difficulty with social skills.

The parietal lobes are well connected to each other. It appears that the relative role of the right and left parietal lobe may change as a skill moves from being initially learned to being mastered. For example, early speech development, involving learning the names of objects and people, uses the right parietal lobe to define the characteristics of what we are seeing, while the left parietal lobe puts a language label on that percept. After the name has been well learned, the left parietal lobe can maintain the skill on its own. There is evidence to suggest that early reading skills—the learning of letter recognition and initial word decoding, involves the right parietal lobe, while later reading skills that require the association of language meaning with words (reading comprehension) involves the left parietal lobe.

Once we move beyond the initial learning of letter, number, and word recognition, the left parietal lobe plays an important role in a child's continued development of academic skills. When seizures disrupt the left parietal lobe, he may have problems with reading comprehension, spelling, and expressing thoughts in writing. The child may have difficulty acquiring the concepts underlying math operations. He may be able to add and subtract when groups of objects are present, but be unable to do these same operations if a parent asks "What is 4 plus 5?" He may be unable to select the correct operation when presented with a story problem.

▶ **What can you do to help your child when seizures involve the parietal lobe?**
It is normal to have skill strengths and weaknesses. We all have things we are good at and things that we are not very good at. When one parietal lobe is not working well, the extent of difference between strong and weak skills may be greater. As a parent, you need to know what skills have been affected so that you can set appropriate expectations for your child.

If visual processing skills affect your child's ability to read facial expression and body language, you can help him by telling him what you are feeling. Your child may not notice that you are looking at him with a stern expression, reflecting your frustration at his failure to follow your command. He may not understand that you are upset until you are very angry and have raised your voice. Both you and your child will feel better if you use words from the start to let him know that commands are important ("I really mean it! Do it now!", "I am angry with you." It makes me sad when you . . . ").

When the right parietal lobe is not working properly, your child may not be interested in sports that involve visual processing such as baseball or basketball. However, she may enjoy sports such as swimming or track. Children with visual processing problems may not enjoy putting together a jigsaw puzzle with the family or may not want to enroll in an art class. Understanding your child's skill pattern will help you to encourage her participation in activities that will provide her with successful experiences.

Problems with visual processing can affect academic work. For example, learning the location of places on a map depends on good spatial skills. You can help your child compensate for visual processing problems by teaching him to use language to "talk about" what he sees. For example, in learning the location of major rivers in the United States, he can describe the Mississippi River as in the middle of the map, going from top to bottom. The Ohio River runs into the Mississippi from the right, the Missouri runs into the Mississippi from the left. Multistep math operations are often demonstrated by the teacher and presented as a series of spatial movements. You can help your child remember this pattern by having him identify a word or phrase to help him remember each step, making a verbal (written) outline of the procedure.

When the left parietal lobe is not working well, your child may have difficulty learning reading, spelling, or writing skills (a language-based learning disability). Your child's school is responsible for addressing her learning needs. You can help your child by being an advocate for appropriate services so that she gets the help she needs. While children are not likely to be viewed as "dumb" if they have sloppy handwriting, children do get teased about being "dumb" if they have problems learning to read. She may be able to find success experiences in the very things we avoided for the child with right parietal problems. She may enjoy sports activities, art classes, crafts, or music classes. Sharing these activities with peers will help peers to understand that she is much more than her reading skills.

▶ **Who will help me to help my child?**

If your child experiences problems with visual processing, your neurologist may refer you to an *occupational therapist* (OT). The OT uses tests to determine what aspects of visual processing are working well, and what aspects are a problem for your child. Based on this information, the OT may recommend therapy to help him develop the weak skills (remediation). If skills cannot be remediated, the therapist can help him learn strategies to compensate for them. She can work with your child to improve handwriting and drawing skills. In some cases, she may recommend that he be taught to use a computer so that he can efficiently produce legible written work.

Occupational therapy services may be available to your child through his school. Often the OT will consult with the classroom teacher, helping her to set appropriate expectations for your child. For example, if he is having problems with visual processing and handwriting, the teacher may be asked to provide your child with a copy of material that other children are copying from the blackboard or to grade his work based on content and not on neatness. The OT may recommend that your child have access to a computer in school for his written work. These accommodations can be made through a 504 plan.

If your child is experiencing problems with social skills, she can get help through a social skills training group. A social skills group will help her in two ways. First, children are taught routines (what to do) and scripts (what to say) for social situations that they frequently experience. The children in the group practice these routines and scripts through role playing. For example, one child may pretend to tease as another child practices what to do when teased. Second, the social skills group teaches your child a "language checklist" to use in understanding facial expression and body language. For example, the group may talk about differences in the shape of the mouth that indicate when someone is happy, sad, or angry. Some schools offer social skills groups run by the school social worker. If your school does not have a social skills training group, you may be able to get this service from a clinical psychologist.

When the left parietal lobe is not working properly, your child is likely to have problems with the development of academic skills, a *learning disability*. He will still make progress in learning these skills, but may need a slower rate of teaching or the use of a different approach to teaching in order for progress to occur. Just as language is used to help them compensate for right parietal dysfunction, visual cues and real life experience are used to help children compensate for left parietal dysfunction. A neuropsychologist can evaluate your child and provide suggestions to teachers regarding how to help him learn. Your child is likely to qualify for special education services under IDEA in the school setting.

Changing Challenges; Changing Age

CHAPTER 8

Epilepsy During the First Two Years

▶ **What do seizures look like in the first two years of life?**

Babies engage in many random movements. Coordination is just beginning to develop. What one side of the body is doing may not match what the other side is doing. Early in life babies have reflexes that are triggered by how they are moved or positioned. Twitches, jerks, staring, and stretching are all part of normal infant behavior. Seizures frequently look just like these normal behaviors. Often when parents find out that their baby is having seizures, they feel badly because they didn't recognize the seizures sooner. Particularly if this is your first child, you are working very hard to be a "good parent." It is natural to think that you should know something is wrong. However, seizures during infancy are hard to diagnose just by watching a baby. Even physicians can make mistakes. Often, a physician needs an EEG to be sure that a behavior is a seizure. Sometimes a video EEG is used. This procedure involves the use of videotaping while your baby undergoes 24 hours or more of EEG monitoring. It allows you to mark the EEG record via a button press when you see the behavior that concerns you.

▶ **How do I know what my baby needs?**

As you get acquainted with your baby, you develop a sense of what she needs. Some cries sound different from other cries. You get a sense of how your baby looks when she is happy and content, and how she looks when there is something wrong. Pediatric neurologists talk about neurologic "soft signs," behaviors or symptoms that let the neurologist know something might be wrong with the nervous system. You develop similar "soft signs" regarding your baby's health and needs. When epilepsy is diagnosed, it may shake your confidence in your ability to read these "soft signs." Don't worry. Your sense of your baby and her needs will quickly return as you become familiar with her seizures and medication effects.

▶ **What can I do to comfort my baby during and after seizures?**
It is natural to want to protect your baby from any discomfort. During the seizure, your child is typically unaware of what is happening. Although you may see your child's body jerk, he is not uncomfortable or in pain. However, there may be things that you can do during a seizure and immediately afterwards to make sure that your child is safe. Your physician will be able to tell you what is important for you to do for your child's type of seizure.

It is unlikely that your baby will remember having a seizure. After seizures, your baby may be upset because he is confused. When a baby experiences sudden body jerks (myoclonic jerks) he may be distressed because he has knocked over the block tower that he was building or dropped the food he was trying to eat. You can help your baby re-engage in the activity (e.g., rebuild the tower, offer a bite of food). Babies operate in the present. If you make his life fine, your baby will readily return to being happy.

Long before they understand words, babies can sense your emotion from the tone of your voice, changes in your facial expression, and the quality of your touch. Comfort your child with the same things that work when other things have left him irritable and upset. Holding, rocking, and hearing a reassuring tone of voice will help your baby feel secure. Your calm calms your child. For toddlers, it is helpful to tell them that they are OK. During the toddler years, you can use a word or phrase that describes what occurs during a seizure (e.g., "jerks, "shakeys") to explain what has just happened. If you can be matter-of-fact (e.g., "That was just one of your jerks."), your child will learn to feel that way about his seizures as well.

▶ **How will I get my child to take medication?**
Your physician and pharmacist will help you get a form of medication appropriate to your child's age. For most babies, liquid forms of the anti-epileptic drugs (AEDs) are used. Your pharmacy may be able to provide you with a bottle stopper that allows you to attach a medicine syringe. This makes it easier for you to get the right dose for your baby while reducing the chance for spills. With a little practice, you and your infant will find a method that works best for making sure the medicine ends up in his mouth and is swallowed. The times that medicine coated your infant's face, went up his nose,

or ended up in your hair will become funny memories. For toddlers, some medications are available as "sprinkles" or can be crushed, then mixed with foods such as applesauce, yogurt, or ice cream. Your toddler may find that this tastes better than the liquid form.

Your attitude when giving medication is important. Remember, your infant can tell when you are tense, tending to become more irritable in response to this tension. So relax. Medicine is important, but you *will* succeed in giving it. Make giving medicine as routine an event as giving your baby a bath or changing a diaper. The more that it becomes part of your baby's routine, the less resistance you will encounter as he grows up. If you approach giving medication in a confident, matter-of-fact manner, your child will be more likely to cooperate.

While most infants take medication well, giving medication can become more challenging as your baby grows into the toddler years. Once children learn to use the word "no," they typically test out the use of that word in many settings. Most parents encounter at least a few times when their child objects to taking medication. However, if this becomes a daily problem, you need to take action to resolve it as quickly as possible. Talk with your neurologist. It may be that a change in medication or in the supplier of a medication resulted in a product that tastes bad to your child. A different form of the medication may work better. If talking with the neurologist does not help, ask for a referral to a pediatric psychologist to serve as a coach in helping you and your child work through this problem.

▶ **How will I find child care while I work or a babysitter so that I can go out?**
Finding good child care is a challenge for all parents. As you interview child care providers, start by asking whether or not the provider has had experience in taking care of children with chronic medical problems. You want to get a sense of the provider's ability to accommodate children with special needs prior to even mentioning the specific nature of your child's needs. Next, inquire about the provider's specific experience with epilepsy. Questions that you may want to ask are summarized in Table 8.1. You want to assess the caregiver's knowledge of epilepsy, her openness to learning more, and her ability to meet your baby's needs. A good caregiver may not necessarily have a lot of past experience with seizures. However, she should be open to learning more about your child's seizures and his special needs.

TABLE 8.1

INTERVIEW QUESTIONS TO USE WITH POTENTIAL CHILD CARE PROVIDERS

1. Have you ever taken care of a baby with any special needs?
   What kind of needs?
   What problems did you encounter with this child?

2. Have you ever taken care of a baby who required medication each day?
   If yes: Where do you store medication?
                  Did you have any problems in measuring the baby's dose?
                  Did you have any problems in giving the medication
                  to the baby?

3. What do you know about epilepsy?

4. Have you ever taken care of a baby who has seizures?
   If yes: Did the baby have seizures in your presence?
                  What did the baby's seizures look like?
                  What did you need to do during and after the seizure?
   If no: Have you every known anyone who has seizures?
   If yes: Tell me about your experience with that person.

4. Are you interested in learning more about my child's epilepsy by talking to my nurse at the neurologist's office or staff from the local Epilepsy Foundation?

5. Are you interested in reading information from my neurologist or from the Epilepsy Foundation to help you learn more about seizures?

6. (For day care center settings)
   What is the adult-to-child ratio for children of my child's age?
   If one child in the group needs individual attention, who is available to supervise the other children?

   (For home child care settings)
   If my child needs your full attention, who is available to help you supervise the other children in your care?

If you have difficulty finding a caregiver for your child, enlist the help of others. If your neurologist works in a hospital-based practice, a social worker may be assigned to the neurology service who can help you. Your county also has a social service department, with social workers who assist parents in meeting the needs of children with developmental disorders. Your local Epilepsy Foundation office may be able to provide you with names of day care centers that have asked for an educational in-service.

To find a babysitter, look for high school students who are interested in health-related careers. These students may be more motivated to learn about your child's special needs. If you live in a community that has a nursing school or a university that awards a degree in nursing, you may be able to find a college student. You may be able to find another mother with a child of similar age who would like to "trade" you some time, taking your child for a few hours with the expectation that you will provide her with a similar break.

Whether you are leaving your child with a day care provider or with a babysitter, you will want to provide her with a fact sheet about your child. This is a good idea for parents to use for any child, whether or not the child has seizures. A sample fact sheet is summarized in Table 8.2.

▶ **How can I help my child if she is slow to develop skills?**
The federal government has passed legislation that requires each state to meet the educational needs of children with learning problems or children at risk for learning problems, the Individuals with Disabilities Education Act (IDEA). A subsection of this act provides funding grants for state administered programs to meet the needs of infants and toddlers who have delayed development or are "at risk" for delays. Names for these early intervention programs differ from state to state. The agency responsible for providing services for very young children also varies from state to state. Your local school system should be able to provide you with this information. Ask to speak to the coordinator for Early Intervention Services. The developmental disabilities section of your County Social Service Department should also be able to help you.

You may wish to start by discussing your concerns with your neurologist. If your baby is having difficulty with the development of motor coordination (sitting, walking, holding objects), your neurologist can refer you to a physical therapist or occupational therapist for evaluation. If your baby does not seem to understand what you say or is slow to learn to talk, evaluation by an audiologist and by a speech and language pathologist is appropriate. These therapists can develop and carry out a treatment program or refer you to the

TABLE 8.2

INFORMATION SHEET FOR CHILD CARE PROVIDERS

Child's Name ———————————— Date of Birth ————————

Mother's Name ——————————— Father's Name ——————————

Place of Work ——————————————————————————

Work Phone ————————————————————————————

Name of Physician ————————————————————————

Office Address ——————————————————————————

Office Phone Number ———————————————————————

Current Medications: ————————————————————————

Medication Name	Time of Day Dose 1	Time of Day Dose 2	Time of Day Dose3
	————	————	————
	————	————	————
	————	————	————

My child takes medication by: ———————————————————

When my child has a seizure: ————————————————————

During a seizure, you will need to: ——————————————————

After a seizure, my child will: ————————————————————

Call for medical help: ————————————————————————

If my child needs emergency medical help,
please take my child to: ——————————————————————

Call parent(s) when: ————————————————————————

My child can do:

———— all the activities that are appropriate for children his/her age

———— all activities but with the following modifications

———— all activities except

Attachment:
Statement of permission to obtain emergency medical care for the child.
Insurance Company
Group Number
Child's ID Number

agency in your community that provides these services. Between birth and three, these services may be provided in your home or day care setting. Besides working directly with your child, the therapists will give you and your day care provider activities to do with your baby between therapy sessions.

▶ **How will I manage my relationship with my spouse?**
The infant years are a challenge for all couples. Every couple goes through a period of adjustment with their first child as they integrate this new life into their relationship. The adjustment becomes more family focused with subsequent children. The introduction of a seizure disorder into the picture tends to prolong the period of adjustment. For every couple with a new baby, the key to adjustment is *communication*. Good communication depends on having time together to talk to one another; time together when you are not too tired to talk. You may need to schedule time together or to call on relatives to help out so that you have the time you need to communicate.

▶ **How can I teach appropriate behavior to an infant or toddler?**
An overview of discipline approaches appropriate for the infant/toddler age range is summarized in Table 8.3.

During the first few months of life, the most important thing that you can do is to bond with your baby—to enjoy, nurture, and love him. Establishing a routine for the baby helps him develop an awake/sleep cycle. When your baby has figured out days and nights, this will be a big bonus to you. Recognize that he will have fussy times for no apparent reason. Once you have checked to make sure that your child is "OK," it is fine to let him cry.

Between 6 and 12 months of age, your baby will gain the ability to move around the room. During this age span, you want to work on helping your child learn to orient to his name. To teach your child to orient to his name, say his name when you are close to him. If he does not look at you, move into his view, and get eye contact with him. Eye contact means that your child is looking at your face as you talk to him. Reach in and stop what he is doing if your baby does not look at you as you call his name. Teaching your child to orient to his name sets the stage for the next step, understanding "No!"

As soon as your baby become mobile (crawling, pulling to stand), begin teaching him to stop what he is doing when you say "No!" in a firm tone of voice. To teach your baby to inhibit to the word "no," you initially need to say "no" when you are close enough to reach in and interrupt what he is doing. By consistently stopping your baby's action and getting him to look at you in response to these words, you are teaching your child to listen to you.

TABLE 8.3

Discipline Approaches for Infants and Toddlers

Behavioral Characteristics:

    Short attention span

    Dependent on others for activities of daily living
        dressing, grooming, feeding)

    Little to no concept of danger

    Little ability to plan ahead or to anticipate consequences of actions

    Egocentric (does not appreciate the needs of others)

    Present-oriented

    Impulsive

    Learning is primarily through experience

    Play is self centered

    Language comprehension is limited

Discipline Approaches:

    Control the environment, reducing the infant/toddler's
        opportunity to misbehave

    Model, encourage imitation of constructive behavior

    Verbally stop misbehavior, paired with physical interruption of behavior

    Direct the child into constructive behavior

    Praise and reward appropriate behavior with parental attention

---

You are also teaching him that you mean what you say. If you say "no," then repeat your "no" many times before stopping your child, your child will learn that he can continue an action and initially ignore you. Your child may play the game of reaching for the buttons on the TV and looking you as you repeatedly say "no" from across the room. The child stops and goes to do something else as soon as you stand up and start to move toward him. You don't want your child to learn that he can wait until you start moving. By immediately interrupting the child's actions as you say "no," you are making certain that if he is heading for something dangerous such as walking towards the street, he will stop when you call his name and tell him "no."

Between 1 and 2 years, children become increasingly able to get into things. At this age, discipline involves interrupting misbehavior, and directing the child into a more appropriate action. For example, if you see your child pulling the cat's tail, you want to tell him "no" to stop the action, then show the child how to pet the cat. At this age, it is equally important to "catch" your child being good. When he is playing nicely, praise him with words or gestures (clapping, giving him a hug, thumbs up). This draws the child's attention to what he *should* be doing. Remember, one goal of misbehavior is to gain parents' attention. If you pay attention to your child when he is behaving, he will have less need to misbehave.

There are also times when it is important to *ignore* a child. Toddlers have temper tantrums, typically set off when the child is not getting his way. Tantrums may involve lots of noise (screaming, crying) and lots of action (kicking feet, hitting, throwing objects, throwing oneself on the floor, head banging). When tantrums occur, you need to make sure the child is safe, and that there is nothing in the way that could hurt him or get broken if he throws it. Some parents place the child in his bedroom, while others simply turn their backs and divert their attention to other things. There are two things to remember when tantrums occur. First, tantrums are designed to get your attention and keep you involved. You need to remove your attention or the tantrum will continue. Second, tantrums are an attempt to get something the child wants or to avoid something that he doesn't want. Giving in guarantees that another tantrum will occur in the future, and the longer you wait to give in, the longer the next tantrum will be.

▶ **How do I ignore my toddler, yet keep her safe?**
Parents worry about their toddler becoming seriously hurt during a tantrum. Parents of toddlers with seizures have the additional concern that their child might have a seizure during or following a tantrum. Ignoring a tantrum means that you are not interacting with the child—it does not mean that you have stopped listening to her, or that you never "peek" to see what she is doing. If your child is headed for danger, you interrupt the action, move her to safety, and resume your ignoring of the tantrum. If she has a seizure, you deal with the seizure as you would at any other time.

▶ **What if my toddler is hitting, kicking, or biting a sibling,**
 a peer, or me?
Children at this age level are learning to regulate their emotions. They are learning to feel "a little" of an emotion, "a medium amount" of an emotion, or "a lot" of an emotion. For example, when happy, a child can smile (a little emotion), can laugh (a medium amount of emotion), or can combine these

reactions with jumping up and down (a lot of emotion). At this age, parents need to help their child learn to appropriately express these variations. Tantrums represent the "I'm mad. I'm frustrated" continuum of feeling. Children in the toddler range need to be taught that physical aggression is not acceptable. We need to be the emotional control that stops the child short of hurting others.

If your child is at the point of hitting, kicking, or biting, you need to immediately intervene with a firm "No!, no hits (kicks, bites)." You can then move her away from others, to a safe place in which to be angry. Be sure to remind the child of what is OK for her to do ("You can hit your pillow." "You can cry and scream.") as well as what she should not do ("You don't bite your sister.") It is most effective to help some children regain calm through use of a "basket hold." For basket holding, you sit on the floor with the child in front of you, then wrap your arms around her body from the back (your leg over her legs if she is kicking). You are giving the child a firm "hug" from behind. In a soft tone of voice, you want to remind her that she is OK, and that it is now time to "calm down."

▶ **What about reasoning with my child?**

Because toddlers are beginning to use language, parents have a tendency to overestimate what a toddler understands. At this age, children are typically able to remember sentences of two to three words in length. They understand words that are concrete in nature, words related to things that they see and experience. Children are aware of their immediate needs, but are just beginning to appreciate that there is a larger social context that influences how and when these needs will be met. The bottom line is that your child is not cognitively ready to understand your attempts to reason with him. Short concrete sentences ("No cookies now. It's not cookie time.") are much more effective than attempts at explanation ("You can't have a cookie now because it is almost time for dinner").

▶ **What about rewards?**

At this age, your attention is the most powerful reward for your child. Hugs, clapping, and smiles are most effective in encouraging your child to repeat a behavior. Other types of rewards require a better appreciation of time and a better comprehension of language than the child has at this age.

▶ **Who can help me during the Infant/toddler years?**

Your neurologist and family physician or pediatrician can help you to know if your baby is developing at a typical rate during these early years. State-sponsored early intervention services will help you and your baby if development is slow. Your family physician and pediatrician may be able to help you develop plans to deal with some of the common behavioral problems that can occur during these years. A pediatric psychologist or child clinical psychologist can help you if behavioral problems persist in spite of your best attempts to address them.

CHAPTER 9

Epilepsy in the Preschool Years

▶ **How do I tell my child about his seizures?**

During the preschool years, children are rapidly learning labels associated with experiences. In the 2- to 3-year age range, it is important to provide your child with a label for his seizures. Children with generalized seizures are unaware that a seizure is occurring, but are aware afterwards that something has happened. They may be confused following a generalized tonic clonic seizure, have dropped things during myoclonic jerks, or missed something during an absence seizure. Giving the event a name related to how the child feels as he regains awareness helps him to understand that something has occurred ("a sleepy", "a jumpy arm"). The child learns to associate the name with the consequences of the event.

Children who have simple or complex partial seizures may be more aware of what is occurring during the event. Parents and children often use names that describe these feelings or actions ("dizzies," "shakies," "the scared"). This helps the parent and child communicate about what is occurring. Using these concrete references to the child's experience is helpful early in the preschool years.

As the child grows, it will be important to let him know that he has seizures that are responsible for these events. Between 3 and 4, you can start to associate the word *seizure* with the child's term for his events ("You had a sleepy seizure. You had a dizzy seizure.") Parents can gradually progress to referring to the events only as seizures. As this term grows in meaning, the child learns to use it as well.

As your child progress into the 3- to 4-year age range, he can begin to understand more about his seizures. Giving seizures a label makes it possible to talk about the treatment for seizures. A child at this age can understand: "You take medicine for your seizures (dizzies, shakies, etc.)." Between 3 and 4 years of age, children are learning about minor body parts (e.g. "ankle, knee, wrist, elbow"). A child with epilepsy needs to be introduced to three important body parts. He needs to know that he has a "tummy" or "stomach" where food and medicine goes. Next, teach your child that the blood moves around his body "soaks up" food and medicine from his tummy/stomach and takes it to all the parts of his body. Teach the child that blood takes medicine to his brain. Finally, teach him that the brain makes his body work and that it also makes seizures happen.

Once your child has learned these important body parts, you can start to explain how epilepsy is treated. The 3-year-old needs to know that medicine helps his seizures (using the child's term for his seizures). The 4- to 5-year-old can understand that medicine goes to the tummy, gets soaked up by the blood, and is carried to the brain to help the seizures. The 3-year-old needs to know that "pokes" (blood tests) tell the doctor how the medicine is working. The 4- to 5-year-old can understand that blood tests show the doctor "how much medicine you have soaked up." The 3-year-old can understand that the EEG tells the doctor "how your brain is working." The 4- to 5-year-old can begin to understand that seizures happen when the brain makes "too much electricity," and that the EEG is checking "the electricity in your brain."

▶ **How can I help my child through medical treatment?**
Children master events in their life, including medical treatment, through their play. Your child will be visiting the doctor more often than most children of the same age. A toy medical kit is a good investment. This allows your child to give "pokes" to her dolls and stuffed animals, check their reflexes, and listen to their hearts. You can make electrodes for your child to use for EEG's on her toys by attaching buttons to strings and allowing her to use tape to attach them to dolls or stuffed animals.

You can use these same play materials to practice medical procedures with your child. When your neurologist orders a medical procedure, ask what will be involved for the child. For example, you and your child can practice having her doll breathe fast or look at a light during the practice EEG. You can make a "tunnel" out of her blocks and practice having a doll slide into the tunnel, lie very still, have a brain picture taken, and then slide back out. While playing with your child you will learn about what she is thinking and feeling.

Children in this age range also master events in their life through story books. Books are available for this age that talk about seizures and the associated medical treatment. Check with your local library or with the Epilepsy Foundation for them. For the 2- to 3-year-old child, make sure that the book has only one sentence per page. For 3- to 5-year-olds, attention has grown so that the child can stay involved with stories that have three or four sentences per page. Once you have a book, read it to your child a number of times. She needs the repetition to gain mastery. Start with two or three times in the first week, then return to the book on a weekly basis for a few more weeks. After that, you can return to the book when the child is about to undergo a medical procedure, or when she indicates a desire to read it again.

▶ **What if my child does not cooperate with diagnostic procedures and treatment?**
If your child is being treated in a clinic associated with a children's hospital, ask to talk with a *child life specialist*, who is trained in child development and in helping children through medical procedures. In the hospital setting, the child life specialist provides play activities for hospitalized children as well as doing "medical play" to help children practice medical procedures. She can give you ideas about how to practice procedures with your child. If you are not in a children's hospital-based clinic, ask your neurologist for referral to a pediatric psychologist.

▶ **Can my child play in the yard?**
In deciding what is safe for your child to do, you first need to consider what would be safe for other children the same age. Most preschoolers are safe playing in a fenced yard. However, no preschool child is safe playing in a driveway or near a street without close supervision. No preschool child should be left unattended while playing in a wading pool or while playing in a backyard with a swimming pool.

Parents need breaks from the constant supervision of their child. Children need breaks from supervision so that they learn independent play and to play with other children. You want to create a safe play area in your house or yard where your child can play alone. If you have only one child, you can purchase safe outdoor play equipment. Look for equipment that is low to the ground or has railings to prevent falls. Anchor equipment in a soft substance that would cushion a fall. Sand or pea gravel not only makes a softer landing area, but also provides opportunities for imaginative play.

When you have more than one child, you will have to set rules for your preschooler. As in any family with older siblings, there are some "no-no's" for the preschool child. For example, there may be a rule that your preschooler can only swing on your lap, or that he may need to swing in a seat-type swing that would minimize the likelihood of falling out. Your child may be able to safely play on monkey bars if you are there to supervise, but may risk falling when you are not there. Be consistent by closely supervising the child at first. Include siblings in reminding your preschooler of limits. He will learn to enjoy the activities that he can safely do when alone.

▶ Can my child play on ride-on toys?

Learning to ride pedal driven toys is important in developing coordination and balance. It is an activity that children do together. Talk to your neurologist regarding what is safe for your child. It may be that a "big wheel," with the seat close to the ground, is safer than a standard tricycle. At bicycle age, it may be important to keep the training wheels on a little longer, providing more stability if the child has a seizure.

Regardless of whether or not your child has seizures, it is important for her to learn from the beginning that she needs to wear a helmet when riding a bicycle, tricycle, or battery-powered toy. Helmets reduce the likelihood of serious head injury for every child (and adult too). Your child will wear a helmet if you consistently enforce that a helmet must be on when riding on things with wheels. It is important that the whole family abide by this rule. You should also wear a helmet, setting a good model for your child. She may enjoy helping to pick out her helmet and decorating it with stickers.

▶ Can my child play with the neighborhood children?

Children learn to play with one another during the preschool years. Each child needs access to play opportunities with other children of the same age to learn and practice these skills. Preschoolers move from *parallel* play (each child playing with the same type of material, but doing his own thing) to *cooperative* play (sharing play materials, assigning roles in the play). The transition from parallel to cooperative play reflects development of the ability to see things from someone else's perspective, a key step in social development. Your child needs play opportunities.

The frequency and timing of seizures will contribute to how you will approach providing your child with peer group play activities. When he is ready to play with others, including going to another child's house to play, you will need to begin your job as an epilepsy educator. If your child has daytime seizures that are not controlled by medication, you may want to start by having other children come to your house for play. If a seizure occurs, you can help the other children understand what has happened. Use the same language for describing the seizure that you use with your child. Other children in this age range want a label for what they saw, and want reassurance that your child is OK.

If your child's seizures are well controlled or happen only in association with sleep, the initial step of being there to teach as seizures occur will not be necessary. Whether seizures are well or poorly controlled, it is appropriate to educate your child's peers regarding epilepsy. You can have a group story time, including your child's books about epilepsy as some of the stories that are read. *Lee, The Rabbit with Epilepsy* is well suited to this age range.

Your job as an epilepsy educator extends to the parents of your child's peers. Even if the child's seizures are well controlled, it is important to let these parents know that your child has epilepsy. Provide parents with a seizure description, describe what you do for him during and after a seizure, and let them know what medication he is taking. A written fact sheet (see Table 8.2) allows the parents to review the information and ask questions.

▶ **How will I find a preschool for my child?**
Many preschool children with epilepsy are developing language skills, intellectual skills, and fine motor skills at the same rate as other children their age. In looking for a preschool for your child, you will want to interview the preschool staff about their experience with chronic medical conditions in general and epilepsy in particular. Table 8.1 provides suggested questions to use in interviewing preschool and daycare staff. Just as you have educated the parents of your child's peers, you will need to provide the teachers with a fact sheet to help them understand your child's needs.

Children with epilepsy are at increased risk for delays in the development of skills needed for succeeding in school. If you have concerns about your child's development, your local school district can provide you with testing to help you know how she is doing compared to expectations for her age level. If your child is showing delays, she is eligible for *Early Childhood Special Education*, a preschool program provided at no cost to you through your school system. Depending on your child's needs, she may receive occupational therapy, physical therapy, and/or speech and language therapy in addition to the classroom program.

The school will develop an Individual Educational Plan (IEP). At this point, re-read Chapter 4, Epilepsy Goes to School, for further information regarding school assessment and the development of an Individual Education Plan.

▶ **What skills does my child have that I should consider in choosing an approach to discipline?**

Important skills developed at this age, and associated behavioral interventions, are summarized in Table 9.1.

At this age, your child makes rapid gains in both the understanding of language and the ability to use language. While she seems like a real little person, keep in mind that her understanding of language remains highly concrete. A child of this age should be able to remember four- to eight-word sentences that involve simple sentence structure. She will be learning language concepts that can be seen and experienced (in, out, under, behind). She cannot yet understand sequencing concepts such as "before" or "after". She will follow the direction in the sequence that steps were mentioned, not in the sequence defined by these terms. For example, if told "Before your brush your teeth, put on your pajamas," she is likely to brush her teeth and then put on her pajamas.

An understanding of time concepts is emerging at a very general level. Your child understands that *now* is not the same as *yesterday* or *tomorrow*. She is beginning to mark time intervals by recurrent events in her day (before or after meals, get up time, bedtime). However, she does not understand the difference between "in a few minutes," "in an hour," or "later this afternoon."

At this age, your child is continuing to learn to regulate emotions. As she plays with others, she is able to enjoy active fun, but is able to stop and settle down if directed to do so. As she develops cooperative play, your child is learning to consider the impact of what she does on others when selecting her actions.

During the preschool years, most children experiment with the power of saying "No" when instructed by parents to do something. Reasoning with your child in an attempt to gain her cooperation through understanding rewards the child with your attention. However, it is unlikely that she will really understand this explanation. Think of the use of "No" as a test to see who is in charge. This is a test that you need to consistently pass.

At this age, you need to start thinking about the difference between a request and a command. A *request* allows the child a choice about whether or not she will do what was suggested ("Do you want to pick up the toys?") When making a request, the child's response of "No" should be respected. You gave the choice, and you need to live with the response. Parents use requests when they know that they do not have the time or are not in a situation in which they could follow through with the consequences of failing to follow the request. *Commands* are statements of what the child is expected

TABLE 9.1

BEHAVIORAL INTERVENTIONS FOR THE TODDLER YEARS

Developmental Characteristics:

    Attention span increases from 5 minutes at age 2 to 15 minutes by age 5

    Language comprehension is improving

    Can communicate wants and needs

    Can anticipate consequences of actions

    Still present-oriented, but is developing a gross understanding of time (an hour is different from a day)

    Feeling word vocabulary includes concepts of happy, sad, mad

    Still egocentric, but becoming aware of the importance of other people in his world

    Parents begin to instruct child in socially appropriate behavior

    Play progresses to parallel play (playing with same type of toys, but each child doing his own thing) and on to cooperative play (assigns roles in plays, shares activity)

Behavioral Approaches

    Time Out

        Behavior based: "Until you are ready to ..."

        Time based: One minute per year of age.

    Contingencies: "If you ..., then you can ..."

    Controlled choices: "It is time to ... Do you want to do either ... or ....?"

    Immediate positive rewards

        Attention

        Praise

        Charts

    Immediate negative consequences

    Checklists (4–5 year age range)

to do. Commands need to be consistently enforced. If you are inconsistent now, your job will be harder in the school age and teenage years. Consistency is a good investment in your child's future behavior.

    Before giving a command, make sure that you have your child's attention.

Children at this age are capable of being engrossed in an activity and may not be listening to you. You want to know that you were heard so that you can set an appropriate consequence if the child does not respond. Keep commands short and straightforward. A choice may follow a command. For example, "Come take your medicine!" is a command. "Do you want to take it with milk or juice?" is a choice. The attached choice helps your child learn to make decisions and gives her a feeling of control in the context of following the overall command. Not every command needs to be followed by a choice.

If your child fails to respond to a command, repeat the command one more time, letting her know the consequence for not complying. Just as a toddler will test to see if parents really mean "No," preschool children test to see if Mom or Dad are really going to enforce a command. If you give in and change your mind, your child has learned that ignoring you is an option. If you enforce the command by setting and enforcing a consequence, your child learns that it pays to do what you say when she is told.

▶ **What kinds of consequences are appropriate at this age level?**
Praise demonstrated through words and gestures remains a powerful tool in helping your child learn good behavior. Catch your child being good. Praise him when he does things the first time you ask. You can start including references to your feelings in the praise ("It makes Daddy happy when you pick up your toys").

If your child does not follow your commands, repeat the command with a consequence (e.g., "Pick up the toys or go to time out!"). *Time out* involves defining a spot for your child (e.g., a corner, a chair, a carpet square in the hallway). Time out can be based on time. As a general guideline, it is appropriate to have the child stay in time out for 1 minute per year of age. Set a kitchen timer. When the bell rings, he is still expected to do whatever you had initially stated. It is important that he follow the initial command before being allowed to go on to any other play activity. If he still refuses to follow the command, time out becomes behavior-based. Your child is not allowed to play until he first announces that he is ready to do what has been asked, and actually completes the task. Parents should continue to check on a regular basis to determine if their child is ready to do what he has been told.

A common problem with the use of time out is that your child will refuse to stay in the time out area. If you have consistently followed through with "no" during the toddler years, a child will be less likely to test your authority when you introduce time out. However, popping out of time out is a good way to gain parental attention. You need to be firm in tone of voice regarding the child's need to stay until the timer rings. The first few times, this may involve sitting behind the child, reseating him in time-out whenever he pops up, to help him understand the concept. Helping your child understand that you will consistently enforce time out is a step towards helping him understand that you consistently mean and will enforce what you say.

Many parents use the concept of "1-2-3 Magic" (see Recommended Reading) to give the child a chance to follow commands. Instead of an immediate consequence, the parent begins to slowly count to three. The consequence occurs when the parent reaches three.

During the preschool years, discipline may also take the form of interrupting misbehavior and guiding the child into a more appropriate behavior. Children at this age can often cite a set of parent rules (Don't throw toys!; Don't bite other children!) However, most children at this age are unable to tell you what they can do when angry. Teaching the "can do" is every bit as important as teaching the "don't do."

▶ **Now that my child is following my commands, what other behavior problems may arise?**

During the preschool years, children continue to learn how to handle negative emotions. While the frequency of full blown temper tantrums may fade, tendencies may persist to strike out when angry or to throw materials when frustrated. At this age, it is important to introduce the concept of "time away." While time out is a negative consequence, *time away* is a positive behavior-shaping approach that helps your child learn to pull out of situations until he regains emotional control. If your child is fighting with siblings, time away may involve sending the children to separate rooms until they are ready to play together without fighting. During time out, the child is not allowed to do anything else. During time away, the child can engage in other appropriate play activities. When an activity is frustrating to a child, he can be prompted to stop, take a breath, and try again.

While toddlers need to rely on behavior to express feelings, preschool children can be encouraged to "use your words" to solve problems. Teaching your child to label feelings is important at this age level ("I'm mad at you"). Your child needs to learn how to ask for help ("Help me"). The use of words to define needs (I'm sleepy. I'm sick. I'm hungry) reduces irritable behavior. Your child learns to use these words by you using them first.

Some children with seizures in the preschool years experience delays in the development of attention and may be hyperactive. Children who are inattentive, impulsive, and distractible need parents to create a structured environment to help them behave appropriately. Structure comes from changing the environment. For example, children who are distractible may spend little time playing with any one toy if all toys are in one large box or scattered around the room. Putting toys in smaller containers (a plastic box for blocks, another box for cars) reduces distractions and helps your child sustain a single play activity. Keeping toys off the dinner table, providing a chair with arms to define boundaries, and a footstool to "anchor" the child's feet adds structure to help him focus on eating.

The hyperactive or inattentive child may need to be told to do things one item at a time so that he avoids getting distracted before all steps of the task are done. Large tasks may need to be broken down into a series of smaller tasks. For example, "Pick up the toys!" may be an overwhelming task, but "Put the blocks in the box!" may be within the child's ability to do without becoming distracted. Consult *Taking Charge of AD/HD* by Russell Barkley for more information on building appropriate behavior in children with Attention Deficit/Hyperactivity Disorder (ADHD).

▶ **What if my preschool age child refuses to take her medicine?**
If your child has had seizures since infancy, the routine for taking medicine that you developed during the infant/toddler years will minimize the likelihood of problems during the preschool years. However, if your child's seizures are diagnosed during the preschool years, you will need to help her to build this routine.

There are four reasons why your child may refuse to take medication.

- The child may not like the taste of the medication.
- The child senses that you don't like the medicine.
- The child does not want to take time away from play to take medicine.
- The child is using taking medicine as a chance to prove that she is in charge.

The response for medication refusal is related to the cause.

If your child does not like the taste of the medication, talk with your neurologist or pharmacist. The same medicine may come in different forms. It may be possible to alter the taste by mixing the medicine with something else, or by changing the type of liquid used to wash it down. If your child is taking liquid forms of medication or having pills crushed and mixed with food, she may do better being taught to swallow pills. The nurse working with your neurologist may be able to help you to help the child practice and master swallowing pills. Since medication can only help the child if it gets into her, it may be necessary to consider a different drug if a solution to the taste issue cannot be found.

When seizures are diagnosed, parents may have mixed feelings about giving medication. While all parents want to help their children, it is natural to worry about side-effects—about how the medicine might change the child. Parents may also feel overwhelmed by the new long-term responsibility of giving medication. A young child will perceive her parent's tension and stress without necessarily understanding why the parent is feeling that way. If you have mixed feelings about treating your child's seizures or questions about administering medication, it is important that you share these feelings with your neurologist. She can address your concerns and allow you to approach your child with confidence.

Giving many of the medications used for epilepsy can be made a part of other daily routines. Some medicines are given with meals, others can be given when your child gets up or as she gets ready for bed. When giving medication is made part of a familiar routine, your child is less likely to see it as "interfering" with her day. If medicine needs to be given at a time of day when your child is usually at play, it is helpful to provide her with warnings that medication time is approaching ("It is almost time for your pills." "Pill time in 2 minutes." "Pill time in 1 minute."). This allows the child to disengage from play. Even though the child does not have a sense of how long "1 minute" is, this routine helps her get ready to take the medicine.

"Time to take your medicine!" is a command. Just like any other command, your child may test to see if you really mean it. While you may be willing to lose other limit tests with your child, you know that this is a command that must be followed. Your child may not appreciate the consequences of failure to take medicine, but you do.

You can reduce the likelihood that your child will test this command by being consistent in enforcing all commands that you give. Your hard work involving being consistent will now pay off. If you have been inconsistent in enforcing other behavioral commands, now is the time for you to change. While the first few weeks may be challenging, your child will learn to listen and to obey your commands.

Teaching your child to follow commands is only part of the answer. You need to make sure that you are giving commands when it is time for medicine. It is easy to slip into "Do you want to take your medicine?" However, your child may be more willing to take her medicine if she feels she has some control. She can be given some control through choices about who will give her the medicine, what the medicine will be mixed with, what drink she will use to wash down the medicine, which pill to take first, or where (in what room) medicine will be given.

Children in this age range will do incredible things to earn a sticker. Doing a daily sticker chart for taking medicine can help to motivate the reluctant child to cooperate. Sharing a fun activity with your child as soon as medication has been taken is also helpful (e.g., "Take your pills and then we can read a story").

If you have tried all of these options and still have not found a solution, there is still hope. A pediatric psychologist can help sort out the reasons for your child's refusals. The pediatric psychologist can then help you and your child to work together to improve compliance with taking medication.

RECOMMENDED READING

Barkley RR. *Taking Charge of AD/HD*, Revised Edition. New York: Guilford Press, 2000.

Moss D. Lee, *The Rabbit with Epilepsy*. Woodbine House, 1989.

Phelan T. 1-2-3 Magic: *Effective Discipline for Children 2-12*. Child Management, Inc., 1996.

ADDITIONAL RESOURCES FOR DISCIPLINE

Forehand R, Long, N. *Parenting the Strong Willed Child*. Lincolnwood, IL: Contemporary Books, 1996.

Mason D, Jensen G, Ryzewicz. *No More Tantrums*. Chicago, IL: Contemporary Books, 1997.

CHAPTER 10

Epilepsy in the Elementary School Years

▶ **How do I tell my child about his seizures?**
If you have used a descriptive term with your child for seizures during the preschool years, it is time to shift from the descriptive term to the accurate label
(e.g., "When you get the dizzies, you are having a seizure.") If your child first
develops seizures during this age range, start out with the accurate term.

Books continue to be a very important means for sharing information
about epilepsy. The memory span for information is still developing at this
age. Children learn through repetition. Books allow you and your child to
return to the information and review it again and again until it is mastered.
Children's books about epilepsy not only provide a description of what is
occurring. The books also provide models for your child regarding how to
cope with his seizures. (See the Recommended Reading in Chapter 4 for
books appropriate to this age range). The Epilepsy Foundation has produced
a pamphlet, *A Child's Guide to Seizure Disorders*, appropriate for this age
range. *You and Your Brain: A Child's Guide* may help both you and your child
understand the relationship of seizures to normal brain functions.

Your physician is an important source of information for your child. Most
pediatric neurologists will be happy to talk with your child about his epilepsy.
Some neurologists have a nurse or physician's assistant working with them
who provides this service. Between physician visits, keep track of your child's
questions, making an "Ask the Doctor" list to take along to the next visit.

▶ **How do I prepare my child for medical procedures?**
Preschool children need to know what will occur. The school-aged child will
want to know both what will occur and why the procedure is being done.

First, you need to understand the "what" and "why" of the medical procedure. There are many sources of information, including your physician, the nurses working with your physician, and the medical personnel who will perform the procedure. If you are in a pediatric hospital-based clinic setting, the Child Life Workers may be able to help you and your child prepare for the procedure. In addition to learning what is involved in the actual procedure, find out if you will be with the child or in a waiting room during the procedure.

Once you understand what will occur, break the procedure down into a series of steps, and review each step with your child. Children in the lower elementary range continue to benefit from "pretend" play to practice the steps. Older children will do fine with a verbal explanation. However, it will be helpful to guide her through the creation of a "checklist" to follow during the procedure to remind your child of the steps. For children in the lower elementary grades, the checklist can be composed of pictures as well as single words. As reading skills improve, the child can identify and record a phrase or sentence for each step as the procedure is described to her.

It is important to be honest with your child. If there is pain involved in a procedure such as a needle stick for a blood test, let your child know that it might hurt. Offer reassurance that the hurt will go away quickly. Let your child know where you will be during the procedure. For some procedures, you will be with your child; for others, you will be waiting close by. Reassure your child that she will be going home after the procedure.

Many parents promise a reward of some sort to their children for cooperating with medical procedures. Rewards can be helpful. The key to rewards is keeping them small and simple. Some children have "sticker books," adding new stickers to the collection with each medical procedure. Rewards can range from a favorite dessert after supper to a visit to the fish tank in the hospital waiting area. Verbal praise ("I am so proud of you.") and hugs can be rewards.

It is important to think about what you promise as a reward. At times, rewards can make it more difficult for your child to get through the procedure. If you promise her that you will stop at the zoo or go to a movie after the procedure is done, she may become so excited about the reward that she finds it hard to "wait" for the procedure to be done. Rewards that are time-dependent ("You will be back at school in time for art class.") can also backfire. In medical settings, procedures are sometimes delayed. If you offer a time dependent-reward, you may not be able to follow through with your promise.

How do I prepare school staff?

It is time for you to review Chapter 4, Epilepsy Goes to School. The first step is to arrange a conference to share information regarding your child's seizure disorder and medication with school staff. If the child's seizures were diagnosed prior to entry into elementary school or during a summer break, contact the school principal in the weeks prior to the beginning of the school year to arrange a conference. In most schools, teachers and administrators are at the school for at least a week prior to the first day for students. The first few days of school tend to be very hectic for the principal and teachers, and trying to communicate this kind of information on the first day of school will be frustrating for both the parent and the teacher. If seizures are diagnosed during the school year, contact the teacher to arrange a conference that includes the school nurse or health aide as well as the teacher.

Contact your local chapter of the Epilepsy Foundation to find out what materials are available that will help the school understand your child's needs. While some schools are very well informed, a lot of inaccurate information about epilepsy is still accepted as fact. When meeting with the school, you will want to get a sense of the school's understanding of epilepsy and experience with children with the same type of seizures as your child is experiencing. If you have any questions about the accuracy of the school's information, you will want to be prepared to guide school staff to good resources.

It is important that you establish good communication with the school. Dealing with a chronic medical condition is a challenge both for the school staff and for you. Because emotions can easily become involved, it is important to make expectations clear at the outset. This includes both your expectations of the school and the school's expectations of you.

How do I prepare my child to deal with peers?

During the preschool years, peers basically want a label for what they see, and reassurance that the child with seizures is OK. During the elementary years, needs for more specific information increase. While kindergarten children will be content with a label and a little reassurance, by third to fourth grade, children want to know the "how's" and "why's" of seizures. The same questions that your child asks you about his seizures are likely to be the questions that his peers will raise. Help your child rehearse answers to these questions. You can do this by role playing. First, let your child pretend to be one of his friends, while you pretend to be the child. Once you have demonstrated things your child could say, switch roles. You pretend to be the child asking questions, while he practices answering the questions. Sharing the Epilepsy Foundation pamphlet, *Because You Are My Friend*, with your child will give him a model of how another child has shared this information.

Teasing is a normal part of life in an elementary school. Every child is teased. Teasing only hurts if a child believes that what others are saying about him is true or might be true. Teasing persists if the child being teased reacts to it, such as becoming upset, crying, or striking out. Talk to your child about teasing, in general terms, before it happens. Ignoring teasing is the most effective intervention for ending it. However, it is hard for children to ignore being teased if they are unprepared for it.

It is tempting to tell your child to tell a teacher each time that teasing occurs. This approach may backfire. Instead of being teased about seizures, your child may be teased for being a "tattletale." If he is being repeatedly teased about his seizures, set up a conference with your child and his teacher to talk about means for addressing the problem. Providing information to peers about seizures may help. While some children will still tease, accurate information may help other children become your child's ally. Classroom activities focused on helping children to appreciate and respect individual differences may help. The teacher or school social worker may be able to identify things your child can say or do to take care of the teasing.

▶ **Besides the school, who else needs to know about my child's epilepsy?**
If every parent of a child with epilepsy educated the child's friends, the friends' parents, the child's coaches, and the child's teachers, the stigma and misunderstanding associated with epilepsy would decrease. However, not every parent wants to be a pioneer with her child.

Many parents approach the task of informing others on a "need to know" basis. Who needs to know? The answer depends on your child's seizure frequency and the timing of seizures. You want to tell any adult that may be responsible for the child when a seizure occurs. If she has seizures during waking hours, this would include parents of children with whom she plays, coaches, and leaders of outside activities (e.g., scouting, church youth groups). If your child's seizures only occur during sleep, you would inform anyone who is responsible for her when she is sleeping (parents of friends where your child spends the night, relatives, camp counselors for overnight camps). If your child's seizures are controlled on medication, the absolute need to inform other adults is less. However, it is important to inform any adult who might be responsible for getting emergency medical care for your child in the event of an accident. Emergency medical personnel need to know that your child is on medication for a seizure disorder.

Even if you don't plan to tell others, you and your child need to practice how to answer questions should they occur. Children in this age range are observant. Peers may see the child taking medication, know that she does not look "sick," and wonder what is happening. Peers may notice that the child has frequent doctor appointments and ask why. Teasing is more likely to occur if your child is unable to answer questions when they arise.

▶ **Can my child take her medication on her own?**
Think about the skills needed to be safe and effective in taking medication. You need to be able to read the prescription bottle. You need to be able to accurately count out the pills. You need to be able to tell time to know when to take the medication. You need sufficient memory to remember to take the medication and to remember that you have taken it. You need to be motivated to take the medication. These skills emerge during the elementary years.

Even for adults, it is important to associate taking medication with some other daily routine (taking it at meal times or when brushing teeth). The kindergarten and early elementary level it is a good time to focus on building these routines. You can start by drawing your child's attention to medicine time in the context of other routines. For example, as the child starts to leave the table having finished breakfast, you stop her and ask: "What do you need to do when breakfast is done?" You want to get to the point that the child will remind *you* of medication time.

If your child does not know how to swallow pills, working on this skill is appropriate by kindergarten age. When medication is taken in liquid form, it is more difficult for your child to become independent in using it. Some parents have used tiny pieces of candy or a small piece of a cookie to practice swallowing pills. Real pills can taste bad as the pill begins to dissolve on the tongue. When this happens, children tend to panic and forget to swallow. Practice with things that taste good to get around this problem. Your pharmacist may be able to provide you with a pill cup that has a ledge for the pill. As the child tips the cup to take a drink, the pill is washed off the ledge and floats down with the liquid. If the child continues to have problems swallowing pills, ask your neurologist or office nurse for further suggestions.

As your child learns to count and label colors, you can start having her count her pills (2 yellow, 1 blue) to make sure that the pills are all there. Once the child can count and can swallow pills, the next step is to buy a pillbox for her. You and your child will initially "load" the pillbox together. Eventually, the child can set up the pillbox, while you check for accuracy when she has finished. Some parents help their child make a color chart so that she can help set out medication by matching to the chart.

Some medications involve a mid-afternoon dose. This is difficult to associate with a routine. By the upper elementary years, your child will be able to use an inexpensive digital watch with an alarm function to serve as a reminder for this dose. You will need to continue to check the pillbox to make sure this dose is taken.

While teaching your child the mechanics of taking medication, it is important to talk with her about the reasons for taking medication. It is easy for a child who is feeling sick to understand that she needs to take medicine to make her feel better. It is more challenging to explain to a child who is feeling well that she needs to take medicine to prevent something from happening. In the preschool years, you have introduced your child to the concept that medicine gets "soaked up" by the blood and that the blood takes it to the brain. It is important to expand on that explanation. Children at this age can understand simple analogies. For example, you can tell your child that the "seizure fighters" in the brain run on the medicine, just like a car runs on gasoline. A car uses up gasoline, so we refill the tank. The medicine is refilling the tank for the "seizure fighters."

Sometimes, medication does not completely control seizures. If your child continues to experience some seizures, reassure her that it is not her fault. Praise her for taking her medication. Remind her that she is helping to make her seizures shorter or to make them happen less often. If the medication has been recently changed, let your child know that medicine does not always work right away. She may need to try the medicine for a number of weeks before the doctor can tell if the medicine will help.

Refusals to take medication occur in this age range. If your child is refusing to take medication, talk to her about her reason for refusal. Unlike the preschooler, children at this age have more descriptive language at their command. Besides issues of taste, children may be able to talk about how the medication makes them feel. Issues of taste and side effects should be shared with your neurologist.

Refusals to take medication may reflect issues of power and control. These are best addressed by providing controlled choices to your child (see Chapter 9 for more information). If problems persist, working with a pediatric psychologist or clinical psychologist is appropriate to address the power and control issues.

TABLE 10.1

BEHAVIORAL INTERVENTIONS FOR THE ELEMENTARY SCHOOL AGED CHILD

Cognitive characteristics

A. Language (verbal description) replaces personal experience as the primary mode of learning.

B. Vocabulary of feeling words increases, allowing the child to express her emotional state more clearly and to comprehend the emotional state of others.

C. Peers become important as behavior models and as reinforcement for behavior.

D. Expectations occur to conform to "social rules" for the sake of others.

E. Time concepts are better understood and impulse control improves, making it possible for the child to postpone actions until later.

Behavioral Interventions

A. Time out (time interval or behavior based)

B. Time away

C. Contingencies (If..., then ...)

D. Checklists

E. Token economy

F. Delayed rewards

▶ How do I address inappropriate behavior?

At this age, children have made the transition from learning based only on what they see and experience to learning through language. Language can be used to bridge the gap between one experience and another. The child acquires concepts to characterize groups of experiences. A key concept acquired during the elementary years is that of time. Children make gains in attention span, impulse control, and memory skills, providing them with the tools to remember rules and to increasingly control their own actions. Improvement in language skills allows them to use language as a coping mechanism—to be able to argue their case rather than tantrum or resort to aggression when frustrated. These skill gains open the door to an increasing range of behavioral interventions.

Time out remains a useful strategy for interrupting misbehavior. With improvement in your child's appreciation of the concept of time, she can be placed in time out for a set period of time. Use of a timer to signal the end of time out remains a good idea so that she will not attempt to negotiate with you about the time interval. Time out can also be behavior-based—the child remains in time out until ready to do what was asked of her.

At this age, your child can also be taught to take "time away." Time away is not a consequence for misbehavior, but rather a chosen opportunity to calm down, or to get ready to do what is asked. For time out, you typically define when the "time out" has ended. For time away, your child controls the interval. Time away is a useful concept for children who find that medication leaves them feeling irritable.

Contingencies ("If you do . . , then you can . . ") and controlled choices ("Either . . or . . ") continue to be useful techniques for children in this age range. Since your child cannot control when a seizure occurs, she may look for ways to have power or control over other aspects of her life. Presenting contingencies and controlled choices allows a child to learn to make good decisions and to experience control, while you continue to exercise judgment about the options provided.

In this age range, charts are often used to track behavior. Charts give a short-term indication of success (smiley face, check mark, stamped mark, sticker). This helps your child bridge the gap from daily behavior to a more long-term reward. Rewards for positive behavior do not need to be immediate. Rather, the child can work over a number of days with the reward provided at the end of the time interval. When charts are introduced, it is essential that the child be given room to improve. If rewards are only provided for perfect behavior, your child may "give up" as soon as she fails to earn a sticker. However, if rewards are based on the expectation of building a behavioral routine, rewards can initially be based on earning only a few stickers, with the criteria for reward gradually increased as she demonstrates competence in the behavior.

As your child masters counting, a token economy can be implemented to support appropriate behavior. She earns poker chips for appropriate behavior, then cashes in the chips to chose from a "menu" of rewards (e.g., a brownie for dessert may cost two chips, rental of a favorite video may cost 10 chips). Your child should be involved in identifying things for the reward menu. By offering both inexpensive and expensive menu items, she will learn about postponing immediate rewards in order to work for a larger reward. While token economies are useful, you need to be aware that they are difficult to manage in a family with many children.

During this age range, attention continues to be a powerful reward.

Prompting appropriate behavior and praising this behavior when it occurs remains an effective management tool. Time alone with a parent to share a favorite activity is often more valuable to a child than a little toy or sticker.

▶ **What should I do when my child has attention problems?**
Attention problems are common in children. Such problems can reflect a delay in the development of brain systems that control attention, concentration, and behavior control. When this occurs, the child is said to have an *Attention Deficit/Hyperactivity Disorder* (AD/HD). Some children with this disorder only have problems with inattention (AD/HD—Inattentive Type). Other children have problems focusing attention and controlling activity level (AD/HD—Combined Type). AD/HD can be treated with medication, environmental interventions, or both. Attention problems can also be a symptom of other problems. Children experiencing depression or anxiety may have attention problems. Delays in the development of language comprehension skills may cause a child to look like he has attention problems.

Children with seizure disorders are at increased risk for AD/HD. This occurs most often when seizures arise from the frontal lobes of the brain. Children with epilepsy are at increased risk for anxiety and depression, resulting in symptoms of inattention. Children experiencing bursts of seizure activity that are too short to be evident as a typical seizure (interictal discharges) may have attention problems. Children experiencing absence seizures will appear to have attention problems as a result of the ongoing seizure activity.

Before you can decide what to do for an attention problem, you need to understand the source of the problem. Problems stemming from anxiety or depression need to be treated with counseling to build more effective coping skills. Adjustments in antiepileptic medications may be used to address absence seizures or the effects of interictal discharges. Providing the child with a work partner (study buddy) can reduce the functional effects of seizure activity on attention in the classroom setting. Treatment by a speech and language pathologist can support the development of language comprehension when language delays present as attention problems.

When attention problems result from a delay in the development of the attention system, environmental interventions can be used to help your child compensate for this delay. In general, children with attention problems do best when provided with structure and routine. You can create structure by setting clear behavioral guidelines in terms of what your child "should do." Routines involve defining a consistent pattern of actions for activities that occur frequently. Routines are typically established for transition times in the child's day such as getting ready for school, getting ready to come home from school, homework time, and getting ready for bed. Your child may need to use a checklist to initially learn the routine. Over time, the sequence of actions will become automatic, reducing the demands on his attention to get the job done.

Environmental interventions may involve physical changes in your child's environment. In the school setting, preferential seating at the front of the classroom can reduce the number of distractions between your child and teacher. It also allows the teacher to use subtle cues such as a hand on your child's shoulder or a light rap on the desk to reorient him if he is off task. At the preschool and kindergarten level, the child may need a placemat or carpet square to define his "spot" for group activities done on the floor. At school and at home when doing homework, restlessness and tendencies to get out of the chair may be reduced by making sure the child's chair has arms and is low enough to allow his feet to touch the floor. Some children with attention problems do best if allowed the option of working while standing. Keeping your child's workspace clear of materials that are unnecessary for the task at hand will reduce distractions. At home, toys may be kept in small containers rather than one large toy box, reducing the tendency to rapidly move from one toy to another.

For some children with AD/HD, environmental interventions are not enough. At this point, it is important for you to talk with your neurologist about stimulant medications. This type of medication can be effective in reducing distractibility. In essence, stimulant medications help a child to keep his attention focused, but do not tell him *where* to focus attention. If your child wants to get school work completed, stimulant medications help keep his attention focused on school work. If the child chooses to focus on something going on outside a classroom window, medication will help him sustain attention to this activity. While stimulant medications may be highly effective, they may have an effect on *seizure threshold*, or the ease with which a seizure occurs. This is why you want to talk with your neurologist before using stimulant medication.

A study by Gross-Tsur and colleagues looked at the likelihood that treatment with stimulant medications would provoke seizures. For the twenty-five children studied whose seizures were effectively controlled with antiepileptic medications, no child experienced a change in control as a result of treatment with stimulant medications. However, among the five children whose seizures were not completely controlled with antiepileptic medication, three had an increase in seizure frequency with the introduction of stimulant medication. All of the children demonstrated the expected improvement in attention in response to the stimulant medications. As with other aspects of your child's treatment, a decision to use stimulant medications is a balancing act, weighing the potential benefits of the drug against the potential risk of a change in seizure control.

▶ **When should I seek professional help?**
All children are learning how to cope with problems during the elementary years. While some children cope effectively, others become overwhelmed. Just like adults, children in this age range can develop anxiety disorders or depression. Unlike adults, children who become depressed are more likely to become irritable and aggressive rather than demonstrate the depression through signs of sadness. If your child demonstrates a marked change in behavior, showing some of the symptoms listed in Table 10.2 and Table 10.3, talk with your neurologist about referral to a pediatric psychologist or psychiatric social worker to help her to develop more effective emotional coping strategies.

Some children have a very difficult time learning social skills. Although most children pick up these skills through everyday play, some need direct instruction to learn to read social cues, and to learn what to say in response to these cues. If your child is having problems making and keeping friends, you will want to talk with school staff about the availability of a social skills training group in the school.

You should seek professional help when you and the school staff have tried what appeared to be reasonable strategies for your child, but the strategies have failed to improve behavior. The school social worker or counselor may be able to give you names of good resources in your community. In addition, most insurance companies have a list of "approved providers" for mental health services. Check with the providers on this list before making an appointment to make sure that the therapist you select has experience with children.

▶ **Can my child participate in sports?**
During the elementary years, recreational and competitive sports leagues are an important source of social activities for children. Most children with epilepsy participate in sports. However, the range of sports that your child can participate in may be limited by the nature of his seizures and seizure control. A child who experiences partial seizures involving loss of control in one arm can not safely engage in gymnastics, where this loss of control could result in serious injury. The same child might be able to play soccer. Talk to your neurologist about what is safe for your child, and talk to your child

about which of these sports might interest him. For some activities, your physician will recommend safety measures. Most often, these measures would be a good idea for any child, including those who do not have epilepsy.

TABLE 10.2

WARNING SIGNS OF DEPRESSION

Irritability, moodiness
Changes in sleep patterns
Difficulty falling asleep
Difficulty staying asleep
Appearing fatigued in the morning
Sleeping during the day
Changes in appetite (either a decrease or increase)
Changes in the child's interest in activities
Withdrawal from activities that the child previously enjoyed
Withdrawal from friendships
Sudden decline in academic performance
Sudden onset of problems with sustained attention

TABLE 10.3

WARNING SIGNS OF ANXIETY

Sudden onset of problems with attention
Sudden decline in academic performance
Reluctance to try new things
Difficulty falling asleep
Reporting of fears
Increased dependence on adults or siblings to be with her
Refusals to attend school
An increase in frequency of body complaints (e.g., headache, stomach pain)

▶ **Can my child stay overnight with a friend?**
If your child would like to go to a slumber party or spend the night with a friend, you need to do a little more planning than most parents. You need to talk to the parent supervising the overnight. If your child's seizures are well controlled, the parent will need to know that your child is being treated for

epilepsy and will be bringing along medication. Depending on the child's age, you will probably want to give this medication directly to the parent rather than having your child keep it with her things.

If your child's seizures are not well controlled, you will want to give the parent a written description of the seizures, including information on what the parent will need to do for her. You want to make sure that the friends who will be with the child know about her seizures so that they will be prepared if one occurs.

▶ **What is my key job during the elementary years?**
During the elementary years, you are helping your child develop the academic skills, behavior control, and emotional coping skills that will help her move from being dependent on you to being an independent young adult. During these years, your job is to provide the opportunities for your child to learn. This includes opportunities to play, to go to school, and to participate with groups of children. It includes building self-esteem through having chores, making decisions, and being responsible for her actions. It also includes opportunities to learn to manage a seizure disorder.

RECOMMENDED READING

Barkley RR, Benton CM. *Your Defiant Child: Eight Steps to Better Behavior.* New York: Guilford Press, 1998.

Barkley RR. *Taking Charge of AD/HD, Revised Edition.* New York: Guilford Press, 2000.

Clark L. *SOS! Help for Parents.* Bowling Green, KY: Parents Press, 1996.

Hallowell EM, Ratey JJ. *Driven to Distraction.* New York: Touchstone Books, 1994.

Humananatomy Board Books. *You and Your Brain: A Child's Guide.* Peapack NJ: Tim Peters & Company, 2000.

Ingersoll B.D. *Attention Deficit Disorder and Learning Disabilities: Realities, Myths and Controversial Treatments.* New York: Doubleday Press, 1993.

CHAPTER 11

Epilepsy in the Adolescent Years

▶ **What do I tell my teenager about epilepsy?**

Adolescence marks the transition from being dependent on parental judgment to trusting one's own judgment. Your adolescent needs all the information that you have about his epilepsy, and needs access to information sources so that he can ask his own questions. Encourage your adolescent to make lists of questions to discuss with his physician, and allow him time along with the physician so that he can ask questions that he may be reluctant to ask in front of you.

▶ **Who do I tell about my adolescent's epilepsy?**

Most teenagers will want to be the one to share the information regarding their seizures, either by telling others themselves or being present when parents talk to others. It is important to talk with your adolescent before you speak to anyone else. Anyone who might be with her when she has a seizure or anyone who would be responsible for getting emergency care for her needs to know about your adolescent's seizure disorder. However, she should have input into how this information is shared. Your adolescent may resist the idea that you are going to talk to others about her epilepsy, but may be more open to helping you develop an information sheet that she can take to these same people. The information sheet for friends should contain a description of the seizure and appropriate "first aid" during and after the seizure. The information sheet for coaches or teachers should include a list of current antiepileptic medications. If the seizures only occur on awakening or during sleep, a simple statement of medications and the fact that seizures occur during sleep may be sufficient.

Some adolescents with epilepsy have had seizures since childhood and peers grew up knowing about the seizures. When seizures develop during adolescence, the issue of informing peers is more challenging. This is a time in life when no one wants to be different. Having epilepsy makes you different. Having what might be viewed as a "brain problem" makes you different in a way that opens the door for teasing and possible rejection. Just as you needed to be an advocate for understanding during the elementary years, your adolescent now needs to take on this role. Teens who have written about the experience of sharing information with peers have described feelings of fear and humiliation as they approached this task. However, once even a few friends knew and understood, teens have indicated that they can then be comfortable being who they are.

Adolescents look to peers to be understood and to suggest ways to cope. Since it is unlikely that your adolescent will have a group of friends dealing with epilepsy, the Epilepsy Foundation has developed resources to meet these needs. In conjunction with the Centers for Disease Control, the Epilepsy Foundation has produced a resource packet, *No Label Required—Teens Talk Straight About Epilepsy*. It contains a videotape in which teens with epilepsy talk about the social problems they encountered and how they approached these problems. The Epilepsy Foundation hosts a teen chat room at www.teenchat.org to allow teens to consult one another. There is adult supervision in this chat room, making it a safe site. Your teen can access "Blurt," a section of the Epilepsy Foundation Web site (www.epilepsyfoundation.org) that provides a link to the chat room as well as personal stories posted by other teens with epilepsy. Your teen can add his own story.

▶ **What new information does my adolescent need to know about his seizure disorder?**

Your adolescent needs to know what *you* know about his seizure disorder. Accurate information is essential so that your adolescent can effectively talk with peers about his seizure disorder. Accurate information is essential so that he can make good decisions about medication compliance. Accurate information is essential so that he can make good decisions about his own behavior. Your adolescent needs to know if specific behaviors might trigger seizures. For example, seizures associated with juvenile myoclonic epilepsy can be triggered by lack of sleep or by the use of alcohol. Fluctuating hormone levels may also be a trigger for seizures. It is known that progesterone has anticonvulsant effects (reduces the risk of having a seizure), while estrogen has proconvulsant effects (increases the risk of having a seizure). Girls with epilepsy may begin to experience seizures related to the timing of their menstrual cycle.

▶ **What does my adolescent need to know about medication?**
Your adolescent needs to understand how medication works. Teenagers feel invincible—they are certain that nothing bad will happen if they take a risk. Medication compliance is a big issue during the adolescent years. Information about how medications are broken down (*metabolized*) in the body and excreted may help your adolescent appreciate the need to replenish her medicine supply each day. Ask your neurologist to explain the dangers of rapid withdrawal of medication (going "cold turkey").

Your adolescent needs to understand possible side effects associated with her antiepileptic drug(s) (AED). Some AEDs are associated with weight gain [valprovate (Depakote®), carbamazepine (Tegretol®), gabapentin (Neurontin®], while others are associated with weight loss [topiramate (Topamax®), felbamate (Felbatol®)]. AEDs can be associated with cosmetic changes such as an increase in body hair, coarsening of facial features, and growth of the gums [phenytoin (Dilantin®)]. Such changes in body image may be a cause for significant distress for your teenager. If AEDs are affecting body image, your teenager needs to share her concerns with her neurologist. He may be able to adjust the dose of the current AED or substitute a different AED without significantly altering seizure control.

Adolescence is a time of emotional turmoil. Some AEDs may help to reduce the likelihood of depressive symptoms, while others may contribute to feelings of depression. Some AEDs contribute to a sense of irritability. While adolescents are known for their hormone-related mood swings, AEDs may play a role in the frequency and severity of these mood swings. Trying to sort out the effects of medication on mood from the effects of being an adolescent can be challenging.

Adolescence is a time when "junk food" becomes much more tempting than mom or dad's home cooking. However, individuals taking AEDs need a diet that is rich in iron to counteract the side effects of many of these drugs. Your neurologist may suggest a folic acid supplement. Some of the AEDs have been associated with osteoporosis in young adults. Since this is an age when you should be building bone density, the neurologist may suggest that your adolescent take a calcium supplement. She needs to know what is being recommended and why.

Your adolescent needs to know that her AED can affect how other medications work. For example, some decrease the effectiveness of oral contraception. Certain antibiotics can enhance or interfere with AED metabolism. While alcohol and street drugs are not appropriate for *any* teen, these substances can be more dangerous for teens with epilepsy.

Teenage girls need to know that antiepileptic drugs can affect the development of a fetus. Information regarding AEDs' effects on fetal development can be accessed through the Epilepsy Foundation Web site, in the Woman's Initiative section. Your teenager can access information about interactions between AEDs and oral contraceptives at this site.

▶ How much responsibility should my adolescent have for his medication?

Your adolescent should be responsible for setting up his pill box and for taking medication each day. As in the elementary years, compliance will be better if he associates taking pills with another routine at that time of day. Your teenager may be able to use extended release forms or AEDs requiring only twice a day doses, minimizing the disruption that taking pills has on his day. If your child has not become independent in taking medication by adolescence, you will want to introduce this responsibility gradually, decreasing the amount of supervision you provide as your teen demonstrates accuracy and responsibility.

▶ What if my adolescent does not take his medication?

If your adolescent was responsible for taking medication independently, missed doses mean that you return to closer supervision. However, it is important to listen to your teenager's reason for missing doses. Your teen may be motivated to take his medication, but may miss doses due to work or school commitments. Your teen may be struggling with side effects that seem minor to you, but are major to him. He may need the opportunity to sit down with his neurologist to talk privately about reasons for noncompliance.

Once you have some understanding of why your teen is not taking medication, you can work together to identify a solution. Teens are more likely to follow through with a solution if they have played an active role in developing the solution.

Let your adolescent know that being responsible about taking medication is the first step to earning other privileges that involve being responsible (going out with a group of friends, dating, a later curfew). Failure to consistently take medication may result in a loss of some of these privileges. Teenagers do well with contracts that spell out expected behavior and the privileges that will result from demonstrating this behavior. Consequences should also be clearly defined. You and your teen need to define what privilege will be lost and how the privilege can be regained. This should be discussed before a problem arises. Putting the contract in writing will greatly reduce arguments if a consequence needs to be enforced.

▶ **Will my adolescent be able to drive?**
It is no surprise to parents that the ability to drive is extremely important to adolescents. If your teenager has seizures during waking hours, most states will not allow her to obtain a learner's permit and driver's license. If seizures occur only during sleep or are controlled with medication, your teenager will need to check with the license bureau to determine if she will be allowed to drive. States differ in the amount of time that a person must be "seizure-free" in order to drive (See Appendix B).

If your adolescent is not allowed to drive, she is likely to view this as a significant limitation to her independence. Some teens rely on friends for rides, while others help out with money for gas in return for rides. Teens can go together with friends and rent a limousine for important events like a prom. If you live in a city with public transportation, provide your teen with opportunities to learn the bus or subway routes. If you drive your adolescent to the library, a movie, or a football game, drop her off at a nearby corner rather than at the front door. If your teen is not allowed to drive, it will be important to let her know that you understand that this is a significant loss. Few teenagers would accept the argument from a parent that driving is just a "little thing."

▶ **What behavioral issues emerge during the adolescent years?**
Teens with epilepsy demonstrate all of the behavioral challenges of teens without epilepsy. However, for the teen with epilepsy, the seizure disorder demands a greater degree of maturity in decision making. It would be good if all teens said "no" to drugs and alcohol. For your teenager, giving into these substances may have far more serious consequences than for the teenager without epilepsy. All teenagers feel that they are invincible, but the consequence can be devastating if the teen with epilepsy extends this feeling to experimentation with missing medication doses or to driving when seizures are not controlled. The challenge of parenting the teenager with epilepsy is to find a balance between your teenager's need for independence and privacy and your need to keep him safe.

All teenagers test limits. You need to be consistent in enforcing consequences. Teenagers need to learn to make decisions. If we don't let them make some decisions, they will never learn how to make a good decision and how to cope with the consequences of a bad one. Effective discipline at this age involves communication with your teenager, arriving at expectations and consequences with input from him.

Teenagers do best with behavioral guidelines that specify what they are expected to do. A list of "don't do's" allows the teenager the defense of "but you never said I couldn't . . . " Any failure to abide by guidelines should be associated with clear consequences. Teens can have input into consequences when guidelines are developed, but should not be allowed to argue for a "lower sentence" once a consequence has been earned through misbehavior. It is essential that you think ahead to the consequences, making sure that you can live with the consequences that you propose. Do you really want to ground your teenager for two weeks? It means that you are grounded too. Make sure that you can handle two weeks with a sullen teenager before using this type of consequence. Tracy's book *Grounded for Life?!* is a good resource to help you to negotiate the challenges of setting expectations and consequences.

Try to identify consequences that are natural and logical. For example, the natural and logical consequence for failing to do homework is a low grade. Failure to put forth effort in all classes results in repeating a grade. Failure to be dependable regarding curfew results in a loss of privileges related to time alone with friends (earlier curfew, a weekend at home). While it is natural for parents to want to protect their adolescents from the "discomfort" associated with natural and logical consequences, it is important to practice "tough love." Natural and logical consequences occur for all of us throughout life. It is better to learn personal responsibility as an adolescent by needing to repeat a class than to learn it as an adult through loss of a job.

Once expectations and consequences are defined, it is helpful to draw up a contract with your teenager. Teens are very good at playing "lawyer," looking for loopholes. A written contract, signed by both parties, allows parents to disengage from these discussions. Although your teenager may later argue with you or complain about the contract, she is counting on you to follow through.

▶ **Are adolescents with epilepsy at increased risk for emotional problems?**
A study by Dunn and colleagues found that 23% of the adolescents with epilepsy surveyed reported the presence of depressive symptoms. Warning signs of depression for adolescents are similar to signs in younger children (See Table 10.2). They found that the type or severity of the seizure disorder

was not a predictor of depression. Rather, risk was associated with the adolescent's satisfaction with family relationships and with his perceived locus of control. *Locus of control* refers to beliefs regarding the role that a person can play in changing what occurs to him. You can help your adolescent feel in control by offering him choices and respecting his decision throughout childhood and adolescence. You can have an impact on your adolescent's view of family relationships by listening to him, considering his opinion, and providing him with responsibilities that will help him to feel that he is a valuable member of the family. All the steps you took to support self-esteem during childhood will pay off during adolescence.

▶ **When is it time for my teenager to leave home?**
Just like teenagers without epilepsy, your teenager will eventually grow into a young adult and want to leave home. You will eventually need to let him go. For some adolescents, the fear of having a seizure away from home interferes with taking steps to living more independently. For teenagers with epilepsy, you need to help them go.

Most teenagers begin the move to independence by getting a job, often during the high school years. In addition to gaining experience in managing the money she earns, the teen builds confidence in her ability to be independent. Depending on seizure control, the teenager with epilepsy may have greater difficulty in finding a job due to employers' lack of understanding of seizure disorders. The teenager with epilepsy may be limited in work opportunities due to her inability to drive. While good for your teenager, holding a job may mean more work for your family in transporting her back and forth to work. Your teen may need your support and an investment of your time to make holding a job a reality for her. Your investment will pay off by growth in self esteem and self confidence.

Some teenagers leave home at the end of high school to go on to college. Some get a job and eventually move into their own apartments. Others leave home when they get married. Teenagers with epilepsy can do all of these things.

Many teenagers with epilepsy have the ability to go on to college. However, they may be reluctant to leave home and live with "strangers" who may or may not understand their epilepsy. By helping your teenager feel comfortable sharing information about her epilepsy throughout childhood and adolescence, you will have prepared her for handling this task on her own.

College entrance exams can be a stumbling block for teenagers with epilepsy. Medications used to treat epilepsy and the effects of the epilepsy itself can contribute to a mild slowing in information processing speed. Since college entrance exams have time limits, this "mild slowing" can result in scores that underestimate your teenager's ability. However, college entrance exams can be taken in an untimed fashion or with more generous time limits if the need for this modification can be documented. Your teenager can get information from his school guidance counselor regarding the documentation required for modifications in test administration. Usually, he will need to have an individually administered intelligence test and an achievement test as well as individually administered measures of processing speed to prove the need for extra time. A neuropsychologist or school psychologist should be able to work with your teenager to gather this information.

Adolescents with learning disabilities are able to attend college. Many colleges offer a Learning Center Program. Special needs identified through testing by a neuropsychologist or school psychologist can be addressed through the Learning Center. This may include interventions such as tape-recorded textbooks, an assigned note-taker in lecture classes, extra time for exams, open book/open note exams, or the use of recognition format testing (multiple choice, true/false, matching).

College is not for everyone. Some teenagers choose to move on to a full time job after high school. Teenagers with epilepsy who are having difficulty finding or keeping a job may be eligible for assistance through vocational rehabilitation services. Each state provides job training and job placement services for individuals with chronic health conditions, physical disabilities, or mental health problems. You can access this service during the high school years by having your teenager talk to his guidance counselor. Vocational training through this service can begin before your teenager leaves high school. Vocational rehabilitation counselors can work with your teenager to identify vocational interests that match your teen's skills. This state-sponsored program can help to pay for further training in order to prepare for employment. This program can provide a "job coach" to help your teenager be successful. Your local chapter of the Epilepsy Foundation may also offer employment assistance.

Sometimes epilepsy is accompanied by significant limitations in intellectual ability. Just because your teenager is functioning in the mentally retarded range does not mean that he needs to live with you thoughout adulthood. Many teens with mental retardation want what other teenagers want, to live independently and to hold a job. As your teenager gets into high school, you will need to begin investigating group home or assisted living resources in your community. You can get information about living and work opportunities for mentally retarded adults through the Developmental Disabilities service section in your county's Social Service Department. The Association for Retarded Citizen's chapter in your area may also be able to assist you. The Association for Retarded Citizen's national Web site (www.thearc.org) can help you locate a chapter in your state or region. Vocational rehabilitation services are available to teens with mental retardation.

▶ **Who will help me during the adolescent years?**
You will continue to have the same resources available to you that you had during the childhood years. Your neurologist and neurology nurse will help you and your adolescent to understand and manage her seizure disorder. School staff will work with you and your adolescent to address special learning needs. The Division of Vocational Rehabilitation, the college Learning Resource Program, or the county Developmental Disabilities section of the Social Service Department will assist you and your adolescent in making the transition to adult living. The difference at this age is that you will be working *with* your adolescent, rather than doing the fact-finding and decision making *for* her.

RECOMMENDED READING

Tracy LF. *Grounded for Life?!*. Seattle: Parenting Press, Inc., 1994.

CHAPTER 12

Some Final Words for Parents

▶ **Can there be quality of life in the face of a chronic medical problem?**
Even though your child has been diagnosed with epilepsy, your family can
still have a satisfying life. There will be moments you will cherish. There will
be times when your child says something that amazes you or leaves you
laughing. There will be times when your child accomplishes something, and
you want to share it with everyone you know. There will be times when your
family has "adventures" together. You will have laughs and have tears. You will
be a normal family, but your definition of what is normal may be a little different from what it is in other families.

Your family will be changed with the diagnosis of epilepsy, as you all adjust
to the unpredictable nature of seizures and the need to make medication
part of a daily routine. Your family may face challenges on many fronts: the
financial challenges of medical care; the additional demands on your time;
the need to learn a new vocabulary for dealing with medical and educational
professionals; the reactions of siblings; and the need to educate others so that
your child is met with understanding.

When faced with change, it is normal to experience grief. Most people
think about grief as something that occurs when someone dies. However,
grief is not restricted to the death of a person. It also occurs when you face
any loss. This loss may be concrete, such as no longer having the money or
the time to do some of the "little extras" that your children enjoyed. The
loss can be more abstract. Every parent has hopes and dreams for their children. A diagnosis of epilepsy can challenge, and sometimes even alter, these
hopes and dreams. Give yourself time to grieve. Recognize that grieving is not
something that you go through in a day, but rather is something that pops

up repeatedly throughout life, triggered by little reminders of old dreams. Focus your energy on the development of new dreams for your child and with your child. There is so much that your child can accomplish. There are so many moments of joy waiting for you and your family. Today may not be one of those moments, but they will come.

As your family adapts to the diagnosis of epilepsy, it is important to focus on providing three "C's" in your family's life: consistency, communication, and compassion.

▶ **Why is consistency so important in raising children?**

Consistency provides children with a sense of security. Children need to know what to expect from their parents. Consistency provides reassurance to your child that you will not let his behavior get out of control. If seizures or medication leave your child feeling "funny," he knows he can count on you to keep him safe during these times. When seizures disrupt family life, consistency provides an overall routine that reassures all family members that each person is still OK.

Inconsistency rewards misbehavior. Imagine yourself at a slot machine in Las Vegas. You put in a coin, pull the lever, and you lose. You try four more times and you win. You are encouraged, and you put in some more coins. After losing five coins, you start to think about quitting, but try a few more coins just to make sure that you aren't still a winner. If it pays off after ten coins this time, you are likely to put in more than ten the next time before considering that you aren't going to win.

Children's behavior works on the same principle. If your child whines, pouts, or throws a tantrum for five minutes and you then give in, you have rewarded this inappropriate behavior. The next time your child does not get her way, she will stay with the negative behavior even longer because it "worked" the last time. If you give in sometimes but not others, your child is likely to persist even longer in the negative behavior because she does not know if it will work.

Inconsistency interferes with the learning of more appropriate behavior. Inconsistency contributes to a sibling's feeling that you are not being "fair." If the child with epilepsy is not expected to do chores and all the other children in the family are, it doesn't just "feel" unfair, it *is* unfair. If the child with epilepsy does not have to obey the household rules for behavior, other children in the family will react with anger to this difference in standards.

▶ **Why is consistency more difficult when a child has seizures?**

Parents often differ in their perceptions of what is fair to expect of the child with seizures. They may have different perceptions of the child's skills. They may have different assumptions about their child's seizure disorder and medication. They may have different access to information sources that would help them understand their child. Often one parent becomes the primary contact for dealing with the child's teachers and doctors.

The seizures, themselves, may disrupt consistency. Expectations appropriate between seizures may not be appropriate immediately after a seizure or during periods of medication change.

▶ **How can parents maintain consistency?**

This leads us to the second "C," *communication*. Parents need to maintain good communication. In today's families, finding time for communication can be a challenge. Both parents may be working outside the home. Children may be involved in after-school activities or need one-on-one assistance with homework. Adding to this busy life, the child with epilepsy may have additional needs for one-on-one help from a parent.

Parents need to make time to communicate. It may be necessary to get a babysitter or relative to watch the children for an hour each week so that you can have some time alone together. This is time to clear the air. This is time to talk about all the children in the family. This is time to share new information about each child, updating each other about school, friends, and medical concerns. This is time to revisit the expectations being set for each child, and to negotiate expectations that you both are comfortable in enforcing.

Parents maintain consistency by supporting each other at the time of discipline. Children quickly learn to whom they should go with each type of request in order to get the answer that they want. Even if you don't agree with your spouse at the moment, it is important to support his or her decision in front of the children. When you are alone together, you can always talk about what you will do different the next time.

Consistency is much easier if you both have the same information about your child. It is hard for both parents to attend every doctor's appointment or school conference. However, it may be possible to use a tape recorder during a school conference. It can help to sit down together prior to physician appointments and school conferences to prepare a list of questions. Some physicians may be willing to talk with your spouse on the phone, or to have your spouse contact the nurse to review what occurred in the visit.

▶ **How do I maintain consistency and communication in the face of divorce?**

Divorces seem to come in two kinds: divorces in which the two parents continue to have open communication; and those in which parents are no longer able to communicate directly with each other. In both kinds of divorce, you need to be clear with teachers and physicians regarding your expectations for sharing information with your ex-spouse. These expectations may be defined legally. The people working with your child need to know what, if any, limits there are on information sharing.

If you have the first kind of divorce, you will need time to do all of the same things that were just described for the two-parent-living-together family described above. If you have the second kind of divorce, consistency and communication must be redefined. It is useful to have an acceptable third party serve as a go-between, ensuring that both parents have the same information about the child. While it is less likely that the child will encounter consistency in expectations between mom's and dad's household, it remains essential that the child experience consistency in expectations within each household. Just as children learn that the school has different rules than home, they can learn that mom's house has different rules than dad's.

▶ **What about siblings?**

As your children grow into the elementary school years, it is important to make time for family meetings. Children need to feel that they contribute to the family, both in terms of doing chores to help one another, and in setting the rules for the household. A family meeting is a good place to review problems that have occurred, and to involve the children in coming up with solutions. Family meetings can also focus on the positive, using some of the time to plan a family activity, or to review the good things that have happened since the last meeting.

The biggest issue with siblings is the issue of "fairness." If your child with seizures also is experiencing developmental delays or learning problems, siblings may need help to understand that he has special needs. This means that the child with seizures may not be able to do all of the things that siblings could do at that same age. You can help siblings to understand that he has expectations that are appropriate to his developmental level. It is important that the child with seizures have rules that are enforced and have behavioral boundaries that he is not allowed to cross (medication may make you moody, but you cannot hit your sister).

If your child with seizures has special needs, contact your library for books written for siblings about your child's unique needs. As siblings approach the teen years, you also need to provide them with ways to explain your child's seizures and any associated special needs to their friends.

A frequent complaint from siblings of children with chronic medication conditions is that they have to "grow up too fast." It is important to set age-appropriate expectations for siblings. In general, siblings should not be left in the position of feeling responsible if seizures occur or an injury results from a seizure. Unless there is a large age difference (preschooler with seizures, high school age sibling), siblings should not be responsible for giving medication or for administering discipline.

▶ **What about compassion?**
The third of the three "C's" is *compassion*. Siblings needs to experience compassion from parents. They need acknowledgment that some things are not "fair." They need to hear that parents recognize that the sibling may feel left out. They need to hear parents acknowledge their right to feel angry if an event that was planned for them was canceled due to their brother's or sister's seizure.

Siblings need a predictable time to communicate with parents about how life is going from the sibling's perspective. For preschool children, this typically occurs through sharing story books and through play. For siblings in the elementary years, this may be provided through nightly "tuck in" time. For older children, this need may be addressed by 15 minutes over an after-school snack, a walk after dinner, or an afternoon every few weeks that is one-to-one time with a parent. In general, teenagers are more likely to talk during a shared activity than if the parent tries to have a defined time to sit down for the sole purpose of talking.

In some instances, a family activity that was previously enjoyed is no longer possible for the child with seizures. For example, it may not be safe to do hike-in, wilderness camping with a child who has frequent bouts of prolonged, generalized tonic-clonic seizures. It is important to find a way to make this activity still possible for the sibling. This can be accomplished by having the sibling share the activity with extended family members, or making arrangements for the child with seizures to stay with someone while the family does this activity.

▶ **Will my family succeed in coping with the challenges of epilepsy?**
Absolutely! Epilepsy becomes part of a family routine. Although seizures are unpredictable, the family will develop a strategy to deal with the seizures

when they occur. Most previously enjoyed family activities will remain a possibility even if they do require a little more planning. The focus on consistency, communication, and compassion is a good basis for any family. The only difference between you and others is that you recognize the importance of these "3 C's" and are putting conscious effort into building them into your family life.

Model Individual Educational Plan For Children With Epilepsy

The goal of the model individual educational plan (IEP) is to provide suggested means for meeting the needs of children with epilepsy. The educational needs for a specific child are related to the characteristics of that child's seizure disorder, including seizure type, seizure frequency, time of day when seizures occur, antiepileptic medications (AEDs), social history, family learning history, and the child's current emotional status. The model IEP provides an overview of potential special needs areas, a means for assessing the skills creating the special need, and suggested programming to help the child compensate for the problems identified. The interventions are provided as suggested approaches to problems. For any given student, school staff may have other, equally appropriate, approaches to assist the student.

Managing the seizure disorder in the school setting

Understanding the Seizure Disorder

- *Goal:* To support the school's understanding of the child's seizure disorder and treatment, parents will be responsible for providing the school with medical information.

    1. Parents will provide the name and phone number of the neurologist and/or nurse clinician caring for their child. An information release will be signed so that an identified school representative can contact the physician/nurse when questions arise.
    2. Parents will provide the school with fact sheets obtained from the neurologist regarding all current AED(s) prescribed for their child. Sheets should include information about frequently observed side effects.
    3. Parents will inform a designated school representative of any changes in medication.

4. Parents will provide the school with a written description of their child's seizure(s), appropriate "first-aid" during the seizure(s), and what the child might need following a seizure.
5. Parents will provide the school with updates if new seizure types develop.
6. Parents and school staff will agree on a system for notifying parents when seizures occur (e.g., phone call, notebook carried by student, tally kept by teacher and sent home on a periodic basis). A seizure record form may available from the local Epilepsy Foundation chapter or the child's physician.

- *Goal:* To reduce social stigma and avoid stereotypes.

1. Teachers will read information provided to them by the parents.
2. Teachers will consult the local chapter of the Epilepsy Foundation for appropriate materials to support education of classmates and school staff regarding epilepsy. The Epilepsy Foundation may be able to offer an in-service workshop for teachers and peers, as well as providing videotapes, information for school nurses, and books or pamphlets for students. If there is no local Epilepsy Foundation chapter, school staff can access information online from the national office at *www.epilepsyfoundation.org.*
3. Attempts will be made to support the child's social development by encouraging inclusion in activities with other children during unstructured times (e.g., lunch room; playground).
4. School staff will consult with the child's physician regarding whether activity restrictions or protective equipment is necessary to allow the child to fully participate in school activities.

Responding to Seizures and Medication Change

Some children may need to change medication or dose during the school year. Medication change is usually done gradually, tapering one medication while slowly introducing a second. During times of change, sedation, seizures, and emotional lability may be evident.

- *Goal:* To support school functioning during medication change.

1. Parents will inform the classroom teacher or school nurse that AED(s) are being changed.

2. The teacher will assess the student's readiness to work through observation of orientation, ability to respond to verbal questions, and ability to generate handwriting during initial classroom activities each day.

3. The teacher will present new concepts in one-on-one or small group settings, getting frequent feedback from the student to check understanding. Title 1 staff (federally funded tutors) may be able to assist teachers in meeting this need at the elementary level. Peer tutors or special education staff may be used to meet this need at the secondary level.

4. If the student seems overwhelmed or frustrated with work related to new concepts, the teacher will provide review work of previously mastered concepts so that the child can remain successful and productive during the period of medication change.

5. When emotional lability (e.g., mood swings) is an issue, the teacher will prompt the student to leave the classroom, or allow the student to leave when the teacher or student recognizes that the student is losing control. A safe area should be identified to which the child can go until he regains control.

6. Parents and school staff will continue to expect the student to complete work assigned even if assignments are modified or she has had to take a break to regain emotional control.

- *Goal:* To manage seizure occurrence in the classroom setting.

    1. The teacher will be familiar with the behavioral manifestations of a seizure, and understand what action should be taken when a seizure occurs.

    2. During the seizure, the teacher will provide reassurance to classmates, responding to their questions.

    3. The teacher will be provided with information by the parent regarding the student's usual functioning immediately following the seizure. If the student is known to experience a reduction in skills in the postictal period (the time immediately following a seizure), the teacher will assess the student's ability to return to work.

        A. The teacher will assess orientation by asking the student to identify the setting, the teacher, and what they were doing prior to seizure occurrence.

B. The teacher will assess language comprehension and processing speed by the student's language output and latency in responding to the above questions.

C. The teacher will assess the student's memory through giving a direction for him to follow appropriate to his usual level of functioning.

D. The teacher will assess motor control through having the student write his name or copy a short sentence. The teacher should observe both the speed and quality of handwriting.

Addressing Skill Weaknesses That May Be Associated with a Seizure Disorder and Medication

Processing Speed

- *Definition:* Processing speed refers to the amount of time required for the child to recognize that auditory or visual information has been presented, effectively assign meaning to the information, and produce a verbal or motor response to that information. Slowed processing speed has been frequently reported in children with a variety of seizure types. While this may reflect the process underlying the seizure disorder, specific medications can contribute to slowing in processing speed.

- *Assessment:* Processing speed can be assessed informally by the teacher and through measures available to the multidisciplinary team.

Teacher Observation:
Observe response latency to questions
Have student produce over-learned written response
(e.g., writing numbers in sequence or letters of the alphabet)
Observe rate of oral reading

Testing Measures
Woodcock Johnson Psychoeducational Battery – III

Reading Fluency	Math Fluency
Writing Fluency	Number Matching
Decision Speed	Verbal Fluency
Rapid Picture Naming	

Wechsler Intelligence Scale for Children, Third Edition
Processing Speed Cluster
Clinical Evaluation of Language Fundamentals - Third Edition
Rapid Automated Naming   Word Classes
Formulated Sentences (observing latency for sentence creation)

Interventions

- *Goal:* To help the student compensate for slowing in verbal processing speed.

  1. Speakers should be aware of their rate of speaking. Inserting brief pauses after key phrases, such as each step in a direction, will allow the student time to process the information presented.
  2. The teacher will provide the student with written instructions to reinforce comprehension of directions given orally.
  3. The student will be allowed to tape record lecture format classes and group discussions for later review.
  4. A designated note-taker will be assigned or the student will be provided with teacher's notes for lecture format classes.

- *Goal:* To compensate for slowing in visual processing speed and written responses.

  1. The student will not be expected to copy material from the textbook or blackboard unless handwriting is the primary learning objective of the task.
  2. The length of assignments will be shortened, reducing the number of rehearsals of the learning objective.
  3. Steps not essential to the learning objectives will be eliminated from assignments.
  4. The student will be allowed to dictate responses to a parent or teacher's aide.

- *Goal:* To ensure that tests provide a fair estimate of ability, all learning will be assessed in an untimed fashion.

  1. For spelling tests, the teacher will tape record the list. This allows the student to pause the tape as she works on spelling each word.

2. Mastery of math facts will be assessed through oral responding, or by number correct with no time limit.
3. If the student has not completed an exam by the end of the allotted time, the student will be allowed to complete it in the resource room, library, or during a study period.
4. Standardized achievement tests will be given in an untimed fashion, or the student will be exempt from such testing. Individually administered achievement tests can be substituted for the group tests to monitor the child's academic progress.

Motor Control

- *Definition:* AEDs can produce tremor, an unsteadiness or shakiness observed in the hands when attempting to write or when manipulating small objects. Attempts to compensate for tremor often slow the rate of work. Tremor can affect the neatness of written work. Seizures originating from brain areas that control movement can result in reductions in coordination that may persist beyond the end of the seizure. In addition, seizures arising from areas involved in visual perception can contribute to poor handwriting and clumsiness on fine motor tasks.

- *Assessment:* This skill can be assessed through classroom observation or by an occupational therapist in the school setting.

Teacher Observation:
> Compare the quality of handwriting when the student is encouraged to work slowly with the quality of writing when the child is working under timed conditions.
> Examine written work for problems with uneven sizing of letters, poor placement of letters with respect to lines, on inconsistent spacing between letters and between words.
> Look for evidence of tremor (shaking or unsteadiness) when the student is buttoning their coat, opening food containers at lunch, or engaging in coloring or cutting activities.

Testing:
> The VMI Developmental Test of Visual Perception—
> Motor Coordination Subtest
> The Developmental Test of Visual Motor Integration

Stanford Binet, Fourth Edition
  Pattern Analysis   Copying
Wechsler Intelligence Scale for Children, Third Edition
  Coding   Block Design
  Object Assembly
Evaluation of visual perception and visual motor skills by an occupational therapist.

Interventions:

- *Goal:* To support work completion, interventions listed above (Processing Speed/Work Completion) will be used.

- *Goal:* To ensure fair evaluation of skills.

  1. The student's written work will be graded on content rather than neatness.
  2. The student will be given oral exams when exams involve essay answers.

- *Goal:* To compensate for impaired handwriting skills.

  1. The student will be introduced to keyboarding skills
  2. The student will be provided with access to a computer for written projects.
  3. A designated note taker will be assigned or the student will be provided with teacher's notes for lecture format classes.
  4. The student will be allowed to use a tape recorder in lecture format and discussion classes.
  5. For students who have learned both printed and cursive letter formation, the student will be allowed to choose the method that is most legible and efficient for him.

Memory
Definition: Memory involves a number of steps. Information is initially held in an immediate memory store, then transferred to working memory for initial processing and action. Long-term storage follows, serving as the basis for building basic information. Partial seizures and epileptiform discharges coming from the temporal lobe may interfere with the initial encoding of

information, while partial seizures or discharges in the frontal lobe may interfere with retrieval. Disruption of attention can also affect the encoding process.

- *Assessment:* The school psychologist or speech and language pathologist can screen encoding and retrieval. If problems are evident, referral to a neuropsychologist for further diagnosis and development of intervention strategies is suggested.

Suggested Measures:
Verbal Memory

Woodcock Johnson Psychoeducational Battery, Revised: Tests of Cognitive Ability
Memory for Sentences   Memory for Words

Woodcock Johnson Psychoeducational Battery, III: Tests of Achievement
Understanding Directions   Story Recall

Clinical Evaluation of Language Fundamentals, Third Edition
Listening to Paragraphs   Concepts and Directions
Recalling Sentences

Wechsler Intelligence Scale for Children, Third Edition
Information   Arithmetic
Digit Span

Visual Memory

Woodcock Johnson Psychoeducational Battery, III:
Tests of Cognitive Ability
Picture Recognition
Wechsler Intelligence Scale for Children, Third Edition
Coding (observe for learning of code)
Auditory/Visual

Woodcock Johnson Psychoeducational Battery, Revised: Tests of Cognitive Ability
Memory for Names   Visual-Auditory Learning

- *Goal:* To support effective encoding of material presented.

1. When directions are given to the class as a group, the teacher will check appropriate retention of the directions by having the student demonstrate what she is supposed to do before beginning independent work.
2. The student will be provided with additional repetition and rehearsal of new information.
3. For rote learned facts (e.g., spelling words, math facts, vocabulary), items will be presented in small blocks (4–6 units), with rehearsal of the block to mastery prior to introduction of another block.
4. Whenever possible, multisensory teaching strategies will be used.
   a. For learning locations on a map, the student will use verbal description talking about the relative position of locations to one another.
   b. For remembering reading material, the student will
      (1) Associate content with pictures in the text
      (2) Make charts summarizing data
      (3) Summarize dates through construction of a time-line
      (4) Stop and take notes after each paragraph
      (5) Create mental pictures of the content of the reading material
   c. To support retention of spelling words, the student will rehearse by:
      (1) Playing Wheel of Fortune or Hangman with spelling words
      (2) Completing multiple choice tests including the correct spelling and misspelled options
      (3) Solving scrambled letter arrays of the spelling word (written arrays or being given Scrabble® tiles for each letter in the word)
      (4) Using phonics to support retrieval of letter sequence
      (5) For encoding problems in the lower elementary years, the student will be introduced to math using the Touch Math system. This system allows for the learning of addition and subtraction operations without the need to memorize all math facts. Provision of a multiplication table to the student will be needed when this operation is introduced.
      (6) For students with severe encoding and/or retrieval problems in upper elementary years, the child will be introduced to a

calculator so that he can progress in work on math concepts even without retention of math facts.

- *Goal:* To support effective information retrieval.

  1. The student will be introduced to multisensory learning techniques (see #4 under encoding) to provide more cues to use in guiding retrieval efforts.
  2. Attempts will be made to relate new material to past learning or real life experiences. By placing new information in a meaningful context, this will provide the student with more cues to use in information retrieval.
  3. Assessment of learning will be conducted through the use of recognition format testing (multiple choice, matching, true/false) rather than reproduction format testing (fill in the blank, short answer, essay).
  4. If a skill has not been used for a period of time, the student will be provided with a guided review of the skill to ensure that the skill has been retained and recalled.

Inattention, Impulsivity, and Hyperactivity

- *Definition:* Inattention refers to a reduced ability, compared to same aged peers, to stay focused on a single speaker or activity until it is completed. Inattention may result from the student being distracted by sights and sounds in the environment or by internal events (thoughts, fatigue, seizures). Inattention may result from a wide range of causes. Children may appear inattentive when they do not comprehend what is said to them. Inattention can reflect organic factors such as those underlying the seizure disorder, or a side effect of antiepileptic medication. Inattention can also be a symptom of emotional distress.

- *Hyperactivity* refers to a level of motor restlessness or movement that is inappropriate for the student's age level. Hyperactivity is often accompanied by impulsivity; that is, responding without waiting for all directions, without developing a strategy for the task, and/or without considering all response options. Hyperactivity and impulsivity may reflect the organic factors underlying the seizure disorder or be side effects from antiepileptic medication.

- *Assessment:* Inattention, impulsivity, and hyperactivity can be evaluated through teacher and parent response to behavioral questionnaires as well as through the student's performance on standardized attention tests.

Parent/Teacher Questionnaires
    Conners Rating Scales
    Attention Deficit Disorder Evaluation Scales
    Child Behavior Checklist

Computerized Attention Programs
    Gordon Diagnostic Systems
    Test of Variables of Attention
    Connors Continuous Performance Test

Other Attention Tests:
    Woodcock Johnson Psychoeducational Battery – III
        Auditory Attention
        Pair Cancellation
    Test of Auditory Processing

Attention, hyperactivity, and impulsivity can be documented through classroom observation. An observer in the classroom watches the "target student" and a peer during at least two different classroom activities. The observer records the time "on task" and classroom behaviors for both students, allowing a direct comparison to "expectations for his/her age." In addition, the school psychologist or special education staff can observe behavior during structured testing.

Interventions:

- *Goal:* Reduction of environmental distractions will be implemented to support attention.

  1. The student will be provided with preferential seating at the front of the classroom and near the teacher. This will reduce distractions between the teacher and child, as well as allow the teacher to use subtle cues (e.g., a tap on the shoulder or rap on the desk) to help redirect the child.

2. The student will be encouraged to keep his desk free of materials that are not essential to the task.

3. The teacher will obtain eye contact with the student, or use touch to orient the student when speaking to him or when giving directions.

4. The teacher will provide an orienting cue to the entire class prior to giving directions ("Class, ready, listen!"). This will help all students in the class.

5. An "office" or study carrel will be provided within the classroom to give the student a quiet place to work. At the upper elementary and secondary level, the student may be allowed to work outside the classroom (resource room, library).

- *Goal:* Attention will be improved in the elementary school setting through the following interventions.

    1. The teacher and student will define a routine for the student to use for checking into the classroom in the morning and for checking out at the end of the day.

    2. The teacher will help the student to develop a checklist to remind her of steps in the classroom routine. When the routine is introduced, the student will be closely monitored in following the routine, given regular prompts, with decreasing frequency of prompts over time.

    3. The teacher will help the student to construct checklists to organize her approach to tasks with multistep directions. The student can use the checklist to help her get back on task if she becomes distracted.

- *Goal:* To support achievement at the Junior and Senior High Level, the school staff will assist the student in developing organizational techniques and study skills.

    1. The student will complete a study skills class that will:
        a. Help the student learn to use an assignment sheet or assignment notebook. In addition to spaces to record assignments, it is helpful for the student to have boxes that can be checked off when work is started on the assignment, when the assignment is completed, and when the work has been turned in to the classroom teacher.

b. Teach the student study techniques that help to focus attention while reading, such as taking notes while reading or reading topic sentences, predicting paragraph content, then reading to confirm the prediction.

c. Teach the student how to break a long-term assignment into daily tasks, then record each task in his assignment notebook.

2. The student will be assigned to "study hall" in the resource room so that the resource teacher can monitor use of an organization system, accuracy of notes and recorded assignments, and comprehension of directions for the mainstream classes.

3. The resource room teacher or guidance counselor will collect weekly reports from teachers regarding late or missing assignments. This information will be provided to parents and student on a weekly basis.

4. For students experiencing organizational problems, the school will provide a second set of textbooks to be kept at home so that the student needs only to take home her assignment notebook and paperwork.

- *Goal:* To help the student compensate for brief interruptions in attention secondary to seizures.

  1. A "study buddy" or work partner will be assigned to help the student find the right book/page, and reorient him to the current topic of discussion or task at hand.

  2. The teacher will check the student's progress during the course of work times, providing reorientation to task when cessation in work is noted. It should be noted that this intervention is equally appropriate for students who are "daydreaming" and for students having subtle seizures. The teacher does not have to make a "differential diagnosis" before helping a student to get back to task.

  3. The student will be allowed to use a tape recorder in lecture classes. The student can review the lecture later, for information that he might have missed.

- *Goal:* To minimize the effects of hyperactivity and impulsivity at the preschool level.

  1. The teacher will use a carpet square, small rug, or placemat to define

the student's "personal space" during group activities that involve sitting on the floor.

2. The student will be seated within arm's reach of the teacher or classroom aide during group activities so that subtle touch can be used to help him stay seated.

3. The school will provide the student with a desk chair having arms to help define limits for movement during desktop activities.

- *Goal:* To minimize the effects of hyperactivity/impulsivity at the elementary level.

1. The student will be encouraged to keep her desk free of all materials that are not directly related to the task at hand.

2. All students will be encouraged to keep writing instruments in their desks until directions are completed and they are told to begin work.

3. The student's schedule will be arranged with breaks between activities that require quiet work and a high degree of concentration to allow the student time to release built up activity. Having the student run "errands" to other rooms, hand out/collect papers, or to take a short break in the gym may be used to help constructively direct the need for movement.

4. Work that is not completed during the assigned time will be sent home for completion rather than having the student complete work during recess. Keeping the student in from recess will only exacerbate the problems with activity level, while at the same time interfering with the child's social development.

5. For some students, it is beneficial to allow them to stand while doing paperwork rather than force them to be seated at their desks.

6. When students frequently interrupt the teacher, the teacher and student will agree on a nonverbal cue for the teacher to use to remind the student to "wait" until she has finished (e.g., a raised hand, palm towards student, signaling "stop").

- *Goal:* To minimize the effects of hyperactivity/impulsivity at the junior and senior high level.

1. The student's schedule will be arranged so that classes requiring concentration and desk work will be interspersed between those that

involve more hands-on work and/or more active physical participation (e.g., art, physical education).

2. The student will be taught to use highlighters to mark places within assignments where directions change to draw her attention to the need to shift directions.

3. Tests will be given in a resource room setting so that the student can be encouraged to check her work before turning in the test. This will also reduce the "pressure" on the student to work quickly and possibly carelessly in order to finish as fast as her peers.

- *Goal:* To support attention and behavior control, the family will discuss the use of medication to address these symptoms with the student's neurologist. It is important for school staff to understand that the stimulant medications frequently used to treat these symptoms may affect seizure control for some children. While medication may be helpful, the use of medication may not be an option for some students with seizure disorders.

Driving and Epilepsy

STATE	SEIZURE-FREE PERIOD (MONTHS)*	PHYSICIAN MUST REPORT?
Alabama	6	No
Alaska	6	No
Arizona	3	No
Arkansas	12	No
California	3–12	Yes
Colorado	No set period	No
Connecticut	No set period	No
Delaware	No set period	Yes
District of Columbia	12	No
Florida	No set period	No
Georgia	12	No
Hawaii	12	No
Idaho	6	No
Illinois	No set period	No
Indiana	No set period	No
Iowa	6	No
Kansas	6	No
Kentucky	3	No
Louisiana	6	No
Maine	3	No
Maryland	3	No
Massachusetts	6	No
Michigan	6	No
Minnesota	6	No
Mississippi	12	No

STATE	SEIZURE-FREE PERIOD (MONTHS)*	PHYSICIAN MUST REPORT?
Missouri	6	No
Montana	No set period	No
Nebraska	3	No
Nevada	3	Yes
New Hampshire	12	No
New Jersey	12	Yes
New Mexico	12	No
New York	12	No
North Carolina	6–12	No
North Dakota	3–6	No
Ohio	No set period	No
Oklahoma	12	No
Oregon	6	Yes
Pennsylvania	6	Yes
Puerto Rico	24	No
Rhode Island	18	No
South Carolina	6	No
South Dakota	6–12	No
Tennessee	6	No
Texas	6	No
Utah	3	No
Vermont	No set period	No
Virginia	6	No
Washington	6	No
West Virginia	12	No
Wisconsin	3	No
Wyoming	3	No

*In many cases, these time frames are modifiable depending on a given patient's circumstances and a physician's recommendation. Information in this table updated as of September 1998.

Index

child psychologists, 31
Child's Guide to Seizure Disorders, A, 107
chores and responsibilities, 26
chronic illness and quality of life, 20-21, 131-132
classmate questions about epilepsy, 34-35
college, 126-129
communication problems (*See* occipital and parietal lobe disorders; speech and oral expression)
compassion, 135
compensatory mechanisms, temporal lobe disorders and, 69
complex partial seizures, 3-4, 25
computerized tomography (CT), 5
consistency in child's life, 132-134
containing behavior, 28
contrast material, in MRI, 6
controlling seizures with medication, 7-9
coping strategies, 28, 135-136
cortical dysplasia, 2

Depakote (*See* valproate)
depression, **118**, 126-127
Developmental Disabilities, 129
diagnosing epilepsy, 1, 4-5
diet, 8, 123
Dilantin (*See* phenytoin)
discipline, 23-24, 29-31, 132-134
    in adolescents, 125-126
    in elementary schoolers, 113-115
    in infant to two years, 89-92, **90**
    in preschoolers, 100-103
disinhibition, 52, 62
divorced parents, 20, 134
drawing/construction, temporal lobe disorders and, 73
driving and epilepsy, 16-17, 125, 153-154
drug use (illicit), 125

Early Childhood Special Education programs, 99
electroencephalogram (EEG), 4-9, 83, 96-97
elementary schoolers, 107-119
    attention problems and, 115-117
    behavior shaping programs and discipline for, 113-115, **113**
    depression and anxiety in, **118**
    examinations and medical procedures for, 107-108
    help for, 117
    learning about epilepsy, 107
    medication and, 111-113
    overnight visits and, 118-119
    parents' role for, 119
    resources for, 119
    school staff and, 109, 110-111
    sports and, 117-118, 117
    telling others, peers, playmates, and friends, 109-111
emotional problems and mood, 28
    in adolescents, 123, 126-127
    anxiety and, **118**
    depression and, **118**, 126-127
    frontal lobe disorders and, 54, 58-59
    irritability as medication side effect, 7, 27, 28
    medication side effects and, 7, 26-27
    temporal lobe disorders and, 66
encoding of memory, temporal lobe disorders and, 71
Epilepsy Foundation, 10-11, 17, 34, 107, 122
epilepsy programs, 10
epileptologists, 10
estrogen, 122
examinations and medical procedures
    for elementary schoolers, 107-108
    for preschoolers, 96-97

facial expression interpretation, occipital and parietal lobe disorders, 76, 77-78

job skills, 128-129
  occupational therapy and, 78-79
  vocational rehabilitation and, 129

ketogenic diet, 8

labeling, 45
learning about epilepsy
  in adolescents, 121, 122-123
  in elementary schoolers, 107
  in preschoolers, 95-96
learning disabilities, 29, 36-39, **38**, 44-45
  in adolescents, 128
  frontal lobe disorders and, 52-53, 59-61
  in infant to two years, 87-89
  occipital and parietal lobe disorders, 79
  in preschoolers, 100-101, 104
Learning Resource Programs, 129
leaving home, 126-129
listening/language comprehension, temporal lobe disorders and, 65, 67, 69-70
locus of control, 127

magnetic resonance imaging (MRI), 2, 5, 9
  preparing for, 6-7
malformation of brain and epilepsy, 45
marriage and divorce, 20
medication, 2, 7-9
  in adolescents, 122-125
  difficulty swallowing, 111
  in elementary schoolers, 111-113
  frontal lobe disorders and, 63
  in infant to two years, 84
  metabolism of, 123
  missed doses of, 124-125
  in preschoolers, 96, 104-106
  refusal of, 104-106, 112-113, 124-125
  side effects of, 7, 10, 26-29, 45, 123

withdrawal symptoms from, 123
memory problems, 45
  frontal lobe disorders and, 54, 59-61
  temporal lobe disorders and, 66-69, 71-72
menstrual cycle, 123
mental retardation, 38-39
mesial temporal lobes, 66, 68
metabolism of medication, 123
migrational disorders, 2
misbehavior vs. seizures (*See also* behavior and discipline; discipline), 23, 24-25
missed medication doses, 124-125
mood (*See* emotional problems)
music, 65
myoclonic epilepsy, 3
myoclonic jerks, 84
myths, misconceptions, stereotypes about epilepsy, 17

neurofibromatosus, 2
neurologists, 10
Neurontin (*See* gabapentin)
neuropsychologic assessment, 9, 43-44
neurotransmitters, 1
No Label Required, Teens Talk Straight About Epilepsy, 122
normal life experience with epilepsy, 18-10

occipital and parietal lobe disorders, 75-76
  body language interpretation and, 76, 77-78
  facial expression and, 76, 77-78
  learning disabilities and, 79
  occupational therapy (OT) and, 78-79
  social skills and, 79
  spatial analysis and, 76
  temporal lobe disorders and, 65
  visual integration problems and, 75-77

time outs, 113-114
toddlers (*See* infant to two years)
tone of voice, prosody and, 65-66, 68, 72
tonic seizures, 3
topiramate (Topamax), 26, 123
transitional scheduling, for frontal lobe disorders, 58
treatment of epilepsy, 7
tremor (shakiness) as side effect, 7, 29
triggers for seizures, 16, 29-31
tuberous sclerosis, 2
tumors as cause of seizuers, 2, 45

unprovoked seizures, 1

vacations (*See also* family activities), 15-16

vagal nerve stimulators, 8
valproate (Depakote), 26, 123
verbal memory deficit, 69
video EEG, 8-9, 83
visual integration problems, occipital and parietal lobe disorders, 75-77
vocational rehabilitation, 129

weight gain, 123
weight loss, 123
Williams, Jane, 18-19
Woman's Initiative, Epilepsy Foundation, 124
word finding difficulties, temporal lobe disorders and, 67-68, 70-71

You and Your Brain, 107